A Colour Atlas of
The Foot
In Clinical Diagnosis

Michael Zatouroff
FRCP Lond., DCH

Physician, Harley Street, London
Honorary Senior Lecturer in Medicine,
Academic Department of Medicine
Royal Free Hospital, London
Honorary Lecturer in Medicine
The London Foot Hospital, London

Lillian Bouffler
DPodM, MChS

Senior Teacher, The London Foot Hospital

Wolfe Publishing Ltd

Copyright © Michael Zatouroff, 1992
Published by Wolfe Publishing Ltd, 1992
Printed by BPCC Hazell Books Ltd, Aylesbury, England
ISBN 0 7234 0813 0

A CIP catalogue record for this book is available from the British
Library.

For full details of Wolfe titles, please
write to Wolfe Publishing Ltd, Brook House,
2–16 Torrington Place, London WC1E 7LT.

Contents

**For
Diana
and
Denis**

Introduction

The foot is usually shod and hidden from view—the body image of this area is suppressed and the physician has little visual knowledge or breadth of data.

There is a place for an atlas to fill this gap and offer the practitioner exposure to more feet than one might see in a year, both normal and abnormal, and of all age groups. Thus this book tries to be a window on looking at feet and assessing the problem while always thinking of the patient as a whole.

> . . . if all be well with belly, feet and sides,
> a king's estat no greater good provides. . . .[1]

This is not a textbook of foot disease nor one of general internal medicine yet it is complementary to definitive texts in both fields. It may be thought to be incomplete.[2] We think that it will be valuable to all health professionals concerned with the care of the feet. The medical and chiropodial student may find all sections of value; those sections specifically describing foot problems will be useful to the practising physician; and the general medicine will be helpful to the practising foot specialist. Social and economic factors and an ageing population make it very cost effective to keep people on their feet, and the elderly and disabled as well as the 'normal' may all benefit from foot care and assessment.

> . . . And Asa in the thirty ninth year of his reign was diseased in the feet, until his disease was exceeding great: yet in his disease he sought not to the Lord, but to the physician.'[3]

The initial chapters cover the first clinical appraisal of the patient as a whole and thereafter the book focuses down on the part of the whole. The range of normal is reviewed—for how can one recognise the abnormal if the normal isn't studied? The later sections are presented as a deductive appraisal from the clinical couch rather than a 'catechism' and take the mind and eye from the foot to the rest of the person.

This structured layout may prompt thought about guided information acquisition and data review. The aim must always be to ask . . . 'Why?'

The photographs were taken by the authors in the normal course of daily work using 35mm single lens reflex cameras with 100mm Macro lenses (Nikon F3/F4—Leica R4/R6) and lit by electronic flash.

[1] si ventri bene, si lateri est
pedi busque tuis nil.
Divitiae poterent regales
addere ma jus.   HORACE. Epistles bk. i epis 12.1.5.
QUOTED BY Montaigne, essays bk. i ch. 42.

[2] '. . . where there is much desire to learn, there of necessity will be much arguing, much writing, many opinions; for opinion in good men is but knowledge in the making . . .' (Milton: Areopagitica).

[3] Asa—King of Judah—died in the 41st year of his reign.
II CHRONICLES 16–12.

MZ, LB
London, 1992

Acknowledgements

We would like to acknowledge, with gratitude, the help of Sir Richard Bayliss, Mr Peter Hamilton, Dr S. Imry, Dr Margaret Spittle and Dr Peter Emerson, who supplied certain illustrations used in this atlas.

1 Looking at the person as a whole

1 **Looking at the person as a whole** — a review of the need to appreciate the normal in order to perceive the abnormal. Feet are attached to people. The patient talks and often discloses the diagnosis. The clues may be in gestures or posture, and though the parts complained about, the bare feet – are offered as a focal point, the extra clues must be looked at, thought about and teased apart.

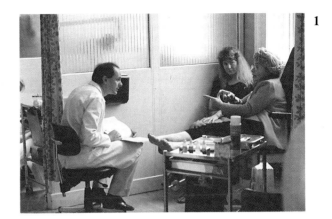

2 **A spider's web.** At first sight that's all it is. But think; let your mind make associations and connections: where's the spider? A train-of-thought association may begin:

- Spider's web→spider naevus→liver disease
- Spider's web→oesophageal web→koilonychia →iron deficiency.

Make associations when presented with a problem. The perception of abnormality requires the recognition of normality (see **3–10**).

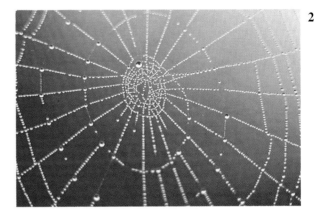

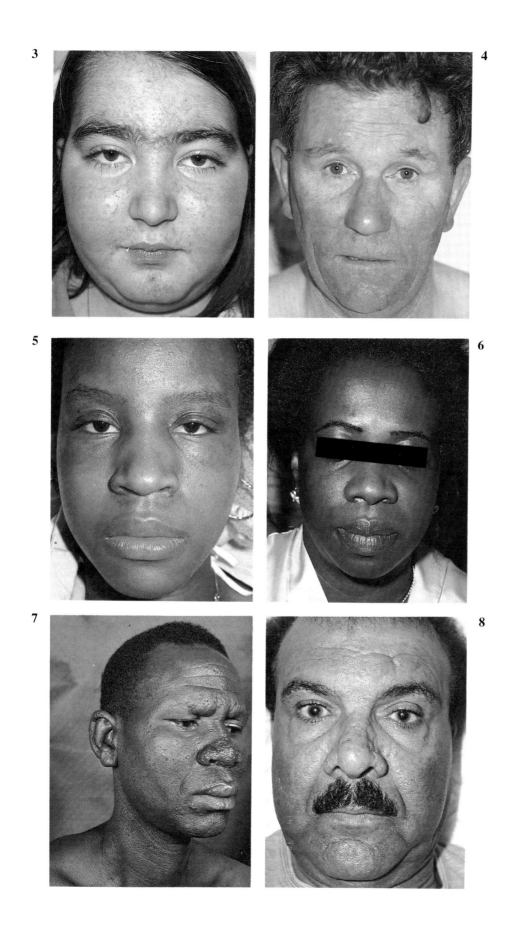

9

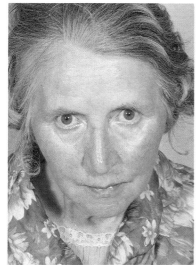

10

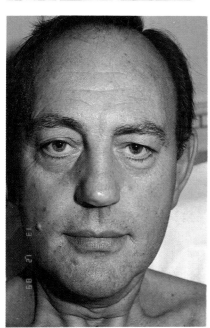

3–10 Facies of disease: can you tell which is the normal one? Compare the *apparent* appearance with the *actual* perception in the following examples.

3 *'Round-faced girl.'* Actually a case of **Cushing's* syndrome—cortico-steroid excess.**

- Round-faced—weight gain
  —salt and water retention
- Acne —blocked sebaceous duct
  —greasy skin
- Hirsutes —excess adrenal androgens
- High colour —thin skin/hypertension.

4 *Facial plethora.* Actually a **healthy outdoor worker.** Facial plethora—normal.

5 *'Two black eyes.'* Actually a case of **dermatomyositis.** A periorbital heliotrope rash on *white* skin, but purple/blue on a black skin.

6 *'Normal.'* Actually a **healthy middle-aged female.** Normal—black dense shiny hair.

7 *'Nigerian farmer.'* Actually a case of **lepromatous leprosy.** Thickened skin of ears and nose. Alopecia of eyebrows—early 'leonine' changes.

8 *'Normal.'* Actually a **normal middle-aged male.** But note:

arcus cornealis – are lipids normal?
old small-pox scars – an anachronism. Smallpox as a disease is extinct.

9 *'Normal intense.'* Actually a case of **Parkinson's†** **disease.** Immobile facies—apparent flat affect and head bent forward by an invisible pillow—sweaty skin.

10 *'Normal.'* Actually a **normal middle-aged male.** Skin over the left eyelid merely lax, not a left-sided ptosis—clearly so, because this fits within the normal database.

The whole is a mosaic whose parts give a clue to the problem. If an abnormality is seen in one part of the body, think of possible causes and look at the whole for clues.

*Harvey Williams Cushing (USA), 1869–1939. Described 1932.

†James Parkinson (UK), 1755–1824. Described 1817.

11

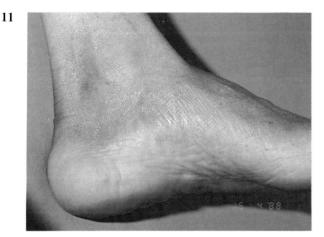

13

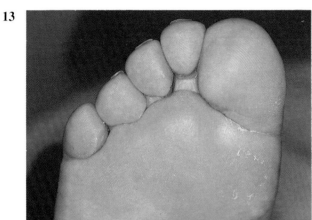

14

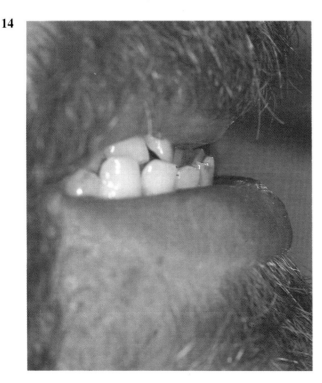

12

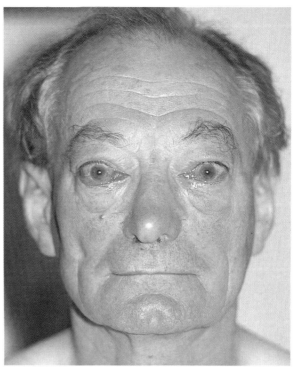

11 Sweaty feet (hyperhidrosis). Common and normal, *or* uncommonly abnormal. Look at the whole.

Causes of hyperhidrosis
- youth
- exertion
- emotion   **OR**
- climate
- fever

Endocrine
- hypoglycaemic
- agromegaly
- thyrotoxicosis

12 The facies of sweaty feet. Thyrotoxicosis—the sweating secondary to an increase in heat production. Note the overall tension, periorbital oedema, chemosis of the conjunctiva and drying at the inner canthus because of difficulty in closing the eyes as a consequence of lid retraction and proptosis (right more than left). The proptosis is masked by the conjunctival injection, so that the clear white around the iris is veiled (compare with **452**). Classic ophthalmopathy of Graves' disease.

13 Big spatulate feet. These could be normal or abnormal, but there is an excess of soft tissue on the pads of the toes, and the tissues of the sole are spilling forwards. The feet sweat a lot, too. All features compatible with growth-hormone excess and enlarging feet.

14 Look at the jaw: **a prognathic mandible and fleshy lip in acromegaly** are clearly evident.

15

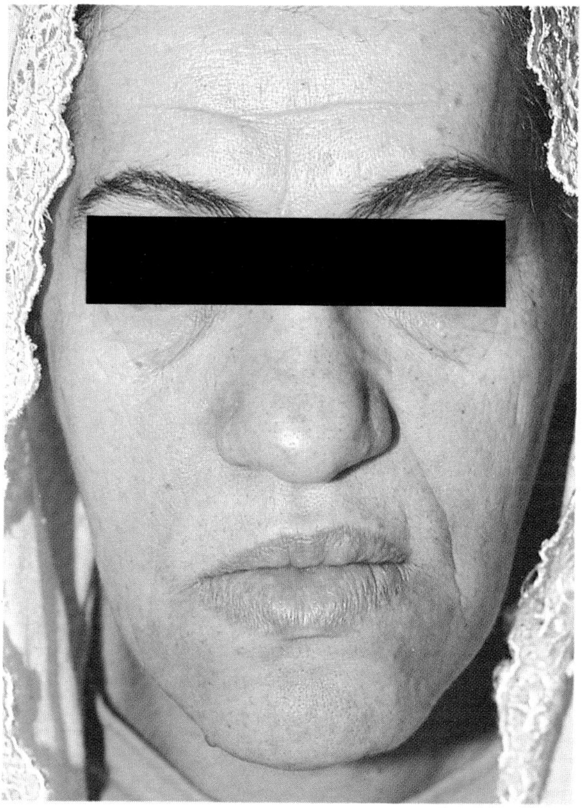

16

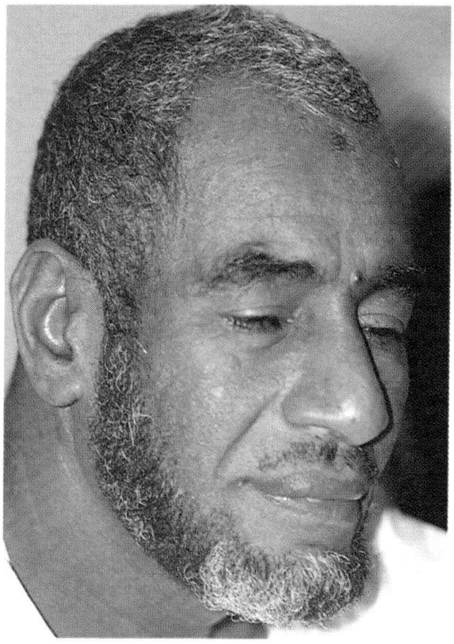

17

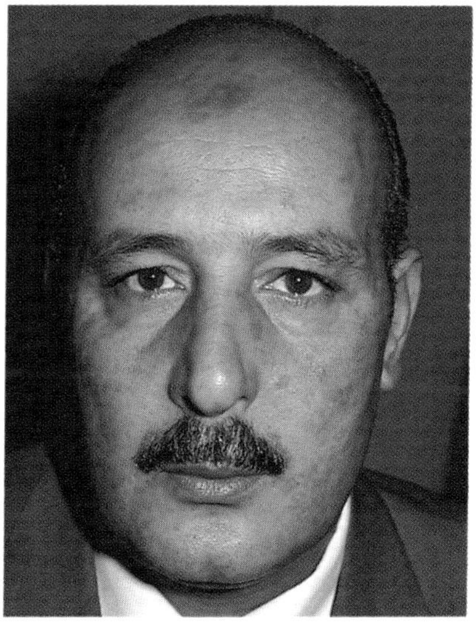

18

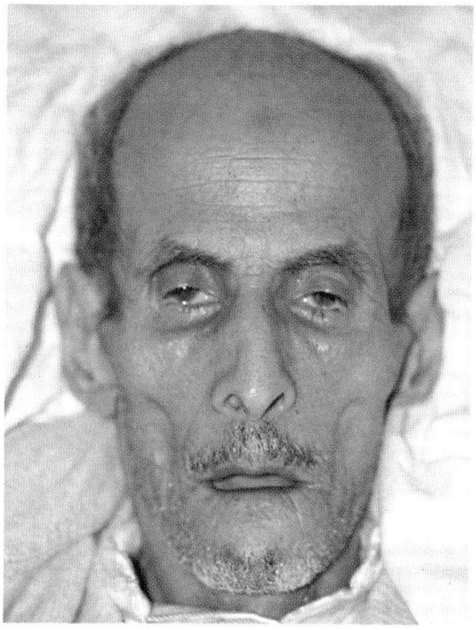

15 The acromegalic face: prognathic jutting jaw caused by mandibular growth; prominent glabellar ridges; increased soft tissue of nose and lips.

Acquire a wide database of normality by looking at people. Notice any deviation from the normal. Then ask: why is it like that?

16–19 The three examples here (**16–18**) all have a mark on the forehead. You realise that the mark is abnormal—but **why?** Having identified it (it's a callus resulting from the physical activity involved in prayer—see **19** on page 12) comment on the significance of the three grades of prominence illustrated here. The first example (**16**) is a clergyman, and the second (**17**) a devout Moslem layman. The last case (**18**) is also devout, but *he* is dying; he is dehydrated, cachexic, and too ill to pray (**18**)—with the result that the the callus on his forehead is actually fading!

Did you note the malar redness across the cheek and nose of the layman (**17**)? Either malar erythema, due to sunlight striking the prominent part of the face, *or* the malar rash of discoid lupus erythematosus.

19

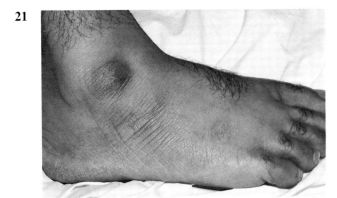

20

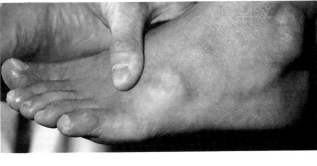

20 The feet. Different cultures sit differently. This patient had a callus over the lateral malleolus from sitting on the ground (as, indeed, did each of the three individuals featured in **16–18** above). However, being an agnostic, he might not have a forehead callus. Note a gouty tophus in the mid dorsal foot, and the ischaemic hairless toes.

21

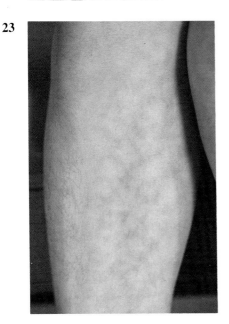

22

23

healed burns at the arrows at each end of the L5, S1 dermatome—deduced even before neurological exam!

23 and 24 Erythema ab igne: pigmentation in the skin caused by chronic application of heat, due to haemosiderin deposition. Found in people who huddle close to a fire or apply heat as a counter-irritation.

Deductions

- Patient feels the cold
- Sits on the left side of the fireplace (**23**)
- Or directly in front of it (**24**)

And

- Has no central heating.

21 and 22 The first example (**21**) looks like a callus over the malleolus from sitting and bearing weight over the bone, but there is another mark proximal to the fourth digital cleft. Examination of the rest of the leg (**22**) reveals a keloid scar, the result of treatment with a cautery in the distribution of the sciatic pain, which explains the

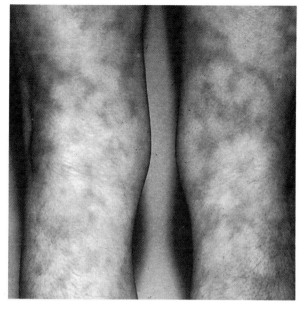

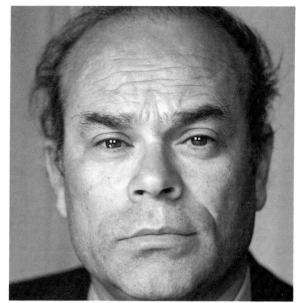

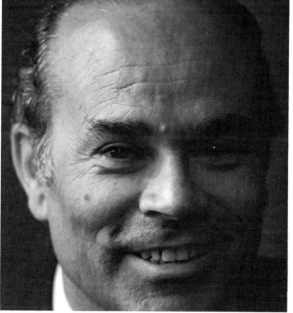

What if no patient is present? Check for clues:
   the bed
   the clothes
   the footwear

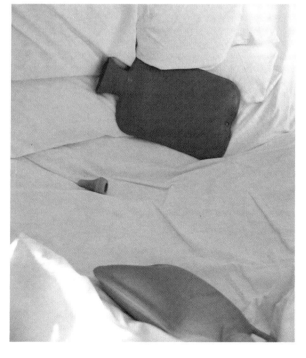

But *why* do such people feel the cold? That must be the next question. Is there a clue? Look at the face (**25**).

25 Appears dull, nondescript, stolid, but feels the cold—odd! Observations lead to further questions: about hypothyroidism, and treatment with thyroxine (**26**).

28 The bed. Two hot water bottles in the bed (i.e. heat as a counter-irritant). The back rest is raised and there is a bell push to summon help—but the patient is in the X-ray department.

Significance

Can you make a diagnosis from the observations (**28** to **30**). The sites of heat for counter-irritation are the small of the back, and the front; the patient prefers sitting—and sitting up. These points can be deduced. So this is a hospitalised patient with pain in the small of the back and in the front, who dislikes lying flat and obtains relief via heat.

The pain comes from the retroperitoneum, and lying flat increases the lumbar lordosis, thus stretching the tissues and aggravating it. A classic picture of carcinoma of the pancreas.

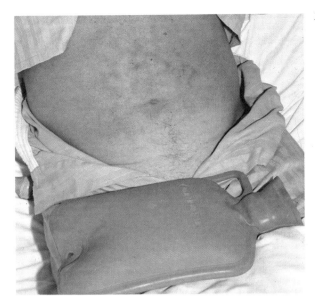

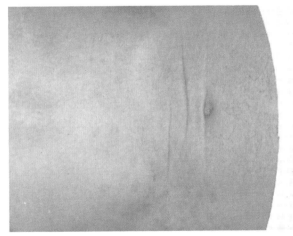

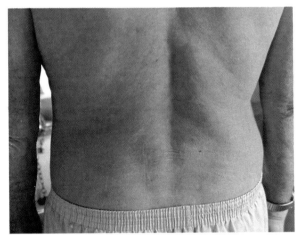

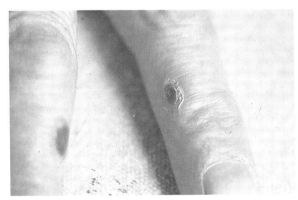

29 and 30 When the patient returns—**erythema ab igne of the belly and back** confirms a clinical (sic) diagnosis.

31 Compare cautery of the abdomen. Heat applied for pain relief/counter-irritation will indicate the severity of the original pain and act as a clue to its site, duration and chronicity.

32 Burns may tell a story. The 1st and 2nd fingers will be touching if they are adducted. Could a cigarette have burnt down as the patient fell asleep—perhaps drunk? Food for thought, at least. Or perhaps the cigarette just stuck to the lip, and the fingers clipped off the glowing tip?

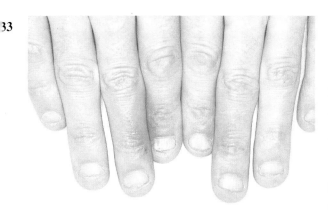

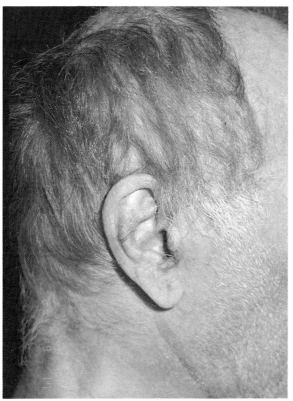

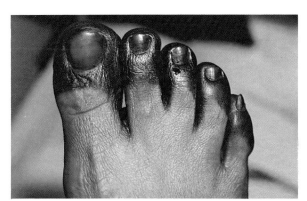

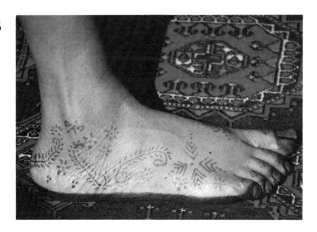

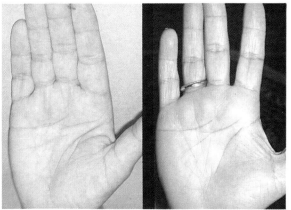

33–37 Cigarettes may stain fingers (**33**), providing a clue to consumption, while bitten nails can be an indicator of stress. Henna will stain the hair (**34**), skin (**35 and 36**) or hands (**37**). It *may* be applied to dye grey hair, but it may also be used for its perceived value in pain relief—the man in **34** presented with headache and tender temporal arteries. Henna on white hair stains red, on black auburn. On palms or soles, it may be used to dry and harden the skin (as in the case of a sailor) for protection from the elements; it may also be used for decorative effect. However, the effect of henna should not be confused with racial pigmentation of the palmar creases or the pigmentation of adrenal insufficiency (right and left, respectively, in **37**).

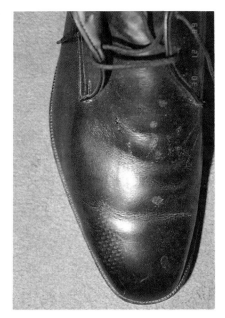

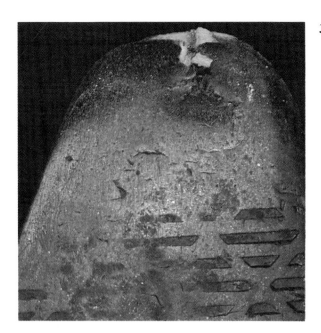

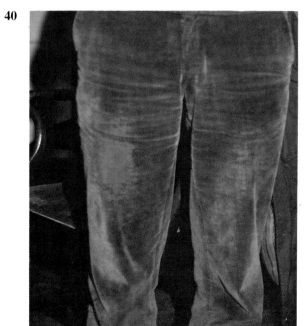

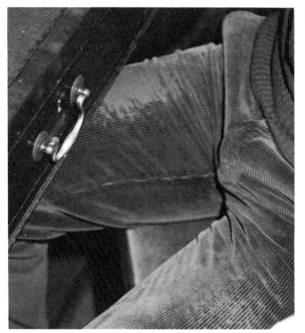

38 The shoes may be showered by urine spray— and if the urine contains sugar, it may dry with a white deposit. If you don't notice the potentially telltale signs in the first place, you may be missing a diabetic.

39 Observe shoe wear: if they are worn at the toe and lateral border, the toe may drag and the leg be circumduct—features of a hemiplegic gait. Such details can be helpful if you want to identify the owner!

40 Observe the wear patterns on the trousers: in this example, they point to the wearer being a right-handed sedentary worker.

41 Deduction is easy once you have noted the wear on the right thigh: this must be caused by friction against a desk, indicating a right-handed wearer who would address the desk by advancing his dominant hand. Try it for yourself: look at the angle of your notebook in relation to the edge of the desk when you are writing.

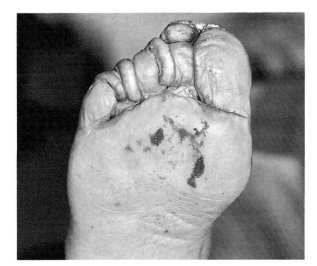

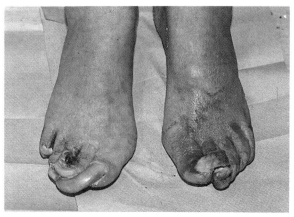

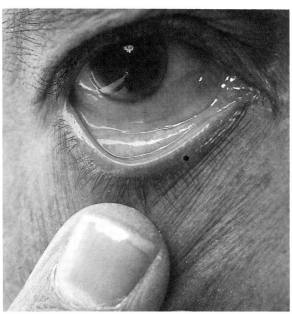

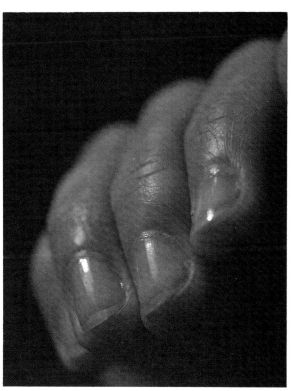

42 and 43 When the shoes are off and the feet are seen to be grossly neglected, again ask why? Is this due to a problem with the whole patient?

The potential medical significance of a neglected foot is considerable. Causes of neglect can include old age, mental and physical disability, alcohol and drug addiction, hypothyroidism, diabetes with the wilful neglect syndrome. Seeing a neglected foot should trigger the question *why*?

44 and 45 If the fingernails are shiny (**44**), it may be a clue indicating the chronic itch of cholestatic jaundice, or diabetes, or malignant disease, or scabies. Compare with the effect of nail lacquer (**45**), where *all* of the nail is shiny—as against merely the tip in cases of chronic pruritis, where the nail is used to scratch the offending itch.

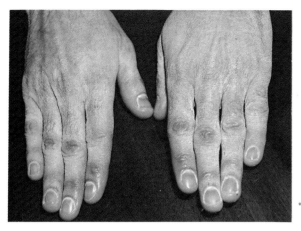

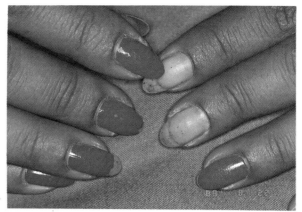

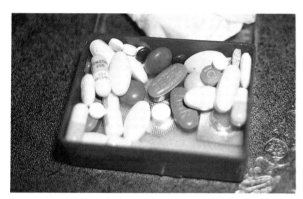

49

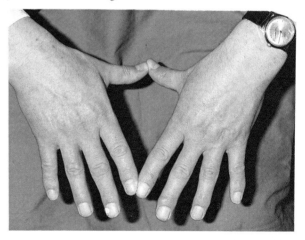

50

46 The hands are dry and defatted—indicators of a chronic obsessive compulsive washer. The patient won't tell you as much, but you should realise the significance of the signs and enquire. Here is a man compelled to wash half hourly and moved to using neat antiseptic as a result of his concern over the AIDS epidemic.

47 Nail varnish selectively chipped and picked off—what can you deduce from this sign? First, the person concerned is obviously left handed, as the nails here are shorter, indicating the *working* hand; also, the varnish becomes chipped earlier and is picked off by the fingers of the right hand, or it is simply picked at as a symptom of stress!

48 Pots of pills. All pills have a message to offer. You can at least hope to get a clue to the symptomatology of the owner, and thus identify the underlying problem or diagnosis. A deduction correctly made may give the patient confidence that he or she has found a perceptive professional.

49–53 Which is the dominant hand—the right or the left? Consider the following examples.

49 The left-handed house painter. Osteophytes at the distal IP joints of the fingers have borne all the wear and tear.

50 The left-handed writer. The callus on the radial side of the left middle finger tells you that this is the dominant hand, but this man preferred to hammer and saw right handed so he wore his watch on the left side!

If the two sides are different, then which is the abnormal side? Often the only way to decide is by knowing what the normal side looks like, and so being able to pick the abnormal side. Sometimes it is not so easy and must be deduced.

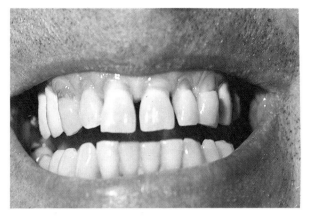

51 The right-handed toothbrusher. Tooth cleaning with a bad technique and a horizontal sawing motion leads to brush abrasion and wear of the tooth on the side opposite to the hand holding the brush, for that is where the force across the curve of the jaw will be strongest.

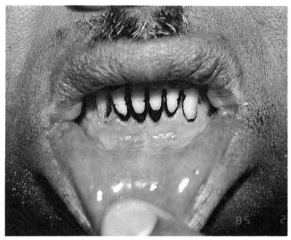

52 The wear is over the right lower canine, but he never cleans his teeth and lodges his chewing tobacco in the buccal sulcus, thus running the risk of induced malignant change.

53

Normal or Abnormal?
If so – which side

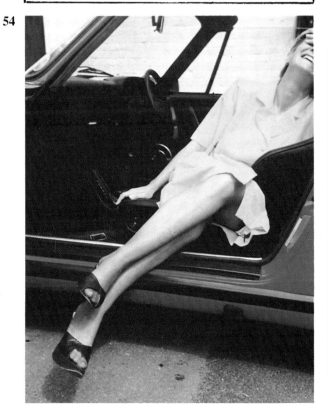

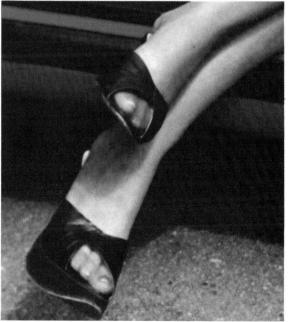

55

for a shortened *leg*? She's attractive to look at, she has good legs, and a red sports car . . . perhaps she is even a little vain? What could be more logical, if she does have one leg shorter than the other, than that she would pose with the damaged leg behind the other leg? The correct deduction is indeed that she has a shortened right leg! Look carefully and you can see.

54 and 55 Pretty girl in a sports car. Her shoes are different—one has a platform sole, the other has not. Has she lost the platform on one shoe by tripping on the pavement, or is the other heel built up as an orthopaedic appliance to compensate

56

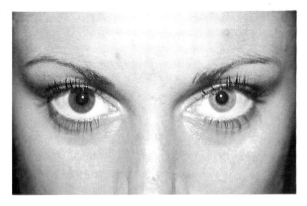

56 Heterochromia. Which eye is normal and which is abnormal? If the difference in colour of the two eyes resulted from the wearing of a coloured contact lens in one of them, then it is more likely that the eyes are both blue, since it is easier to make a blue eye brown than *vice versa*. Alternatively, the blue eye could have been the victim of recurrent uveitis, which could have resulted in the colour falling out; such a situation would predispose to cataracts in later life. There is no ptosis on the left so it is not a perinatal sympathetic Horner's* syndrome.

57

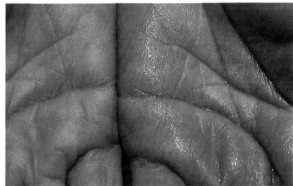

57 Hyperhidrosis. Is the variation here due to an abnormality? If so, which is the 'normal' hand? The hands are hyperhidrotic: as a child, the patient had used his right—dominant—hand in arithmetic classes at school to write on a slate with chalk, but although he always put down the correct answer his sweat erased the chalked solution, leading to the teacher's anger. The pupil thus learnt to have two slates. When he grew up and came to live in England and work as a chartered accountant, his hand still sweated in the act of writing; so he underwent a sympathectomy to produce a 'dry' hand—leaving the other hand, the original 'normal' one, still sweaty!

58

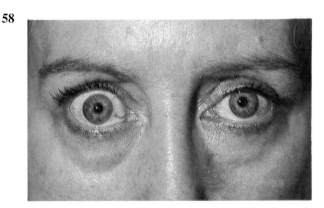

58 Proptosis or ptosis? The patient says that her husband has noted a drooping of her left eyelid. In fact, *the eye complained of* is the normal one, its eyelid's 'drooping' appearance being merely in contrast to the lid retraction affecting the other eye and caused by thyrotoxic eye disease. The trained observer knows which is the abnormal side from long study of normality.

59

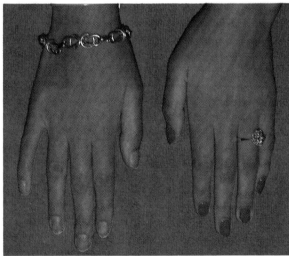

59 Unilateral nail polish. Why would one hand be perfectly lacquered and the other naked? The patient had a cerebrovascular accident and a hemiplegia while on the contraceptive pill. So the manicured hand must be on the patient's paralysed side (unless she has a lady's maid!).

Johann Friedrich Horner (Swiss), ophthalmologist, 1831–1886. Described 1862.

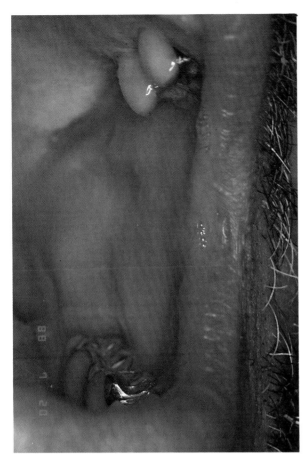

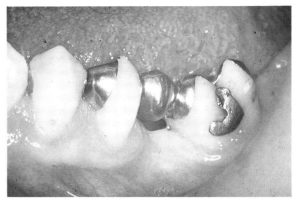

60–63 What of other interesting areas where examination and appreciation may help in understanding a problem?

60 The state of the bank balance from examination of the mouth. It is so easy to look at a patient and not *see*. The immediate impression here is simply of amalgam and gold fillings—nothing to stimulate thought, apparently. But a second look reveals that the gold is very expensive and the amalgam cheap: the patient is on the financial 'up' gradient, but was not always affluent. Now, he can afford expensive, longer-lasting gold inlays.

61 By contrast to **60**, this beautiful technical gold work must have been done by an expert—and cost the earth! But the patient may then have fallen on hard times, for the grotty amalgam *must* have been inserted later by an unskilled worker, for the original expert would never have left such a blemish to mar his work!

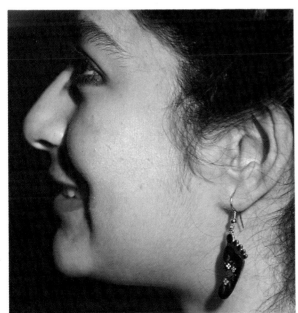

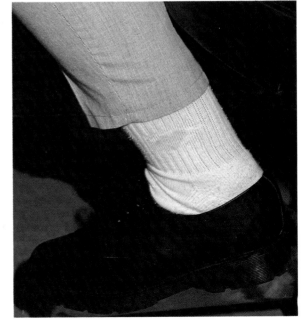

62 and 63 From the 'foot' ear-ring worn in **62**, and the sartorial taste exhibited in **63** ('naturally wearing one's heart on one's socks!'), it is clear that both subjects have to be chiropodists.

64 and 65 Clinical stories from observations of the feet.

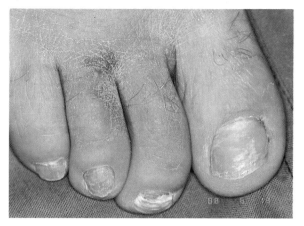

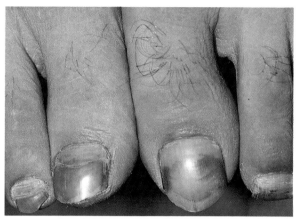

64 Onycholysis in a young male ballet dancer. The nail plate is full of fungus—odd; intractable to treatment (but this is not unusual). However, as well as rampant fungal infections this young man has two areas of purulent folliculitis on the second and third toes—strange. A young male with two forms of infection suggests a defect in his immune system. What is the dark red plaque in the space between the second and third toes, and why is the skin so dry? Clearly (?), Kaposi's* sarcoma and dry skin in the Acquired Immuno Deficiency Syndrome (AIDS).

65 Henna and abnormal skin appendages. Both feet have pigmented nails due to the application of henna—about 7 weeks ago (toe nails grow about 0.5–1mm a week). At that time he ceased applying henna to both feet—why? On the right, there is a growth arrest line (Beau's† line)—these occur if there is a systemic or local upset to the patient. Clearly, being unilateral this upset was local, for though the subject was ill (no interest in henna) the problem was confined to the right leg (see the impaired local growth of nail and the decreased hair growth on that side). An ischaemic problem caused by an embolus of the right popliteal artery.

THE APPRECIATION OF ABNORMALITY REQUIRES THE RECOGNITION OF NORMALITY
INCREASE YOUR NORMAL DATABASE

'They heard because they were condemned to silence, And learnt to see because they had no light'

'The Lucky Marriage' –
Thomas Blackburn (1916–   )

The word with the greatest candle power is 'WHY' (. . . is it like that)?

*Moritz Kaposi–Kohn (Hungarian), dermatologist 1837–1902. Described 1872.

†Honoré Simon Beau (French), 1806–1865.

2 Looking at the feet as part of the whole person[1]

Looking at feet should begin with looking at the patient as a whole. Body weight, size and proportion, the way a person moves, stands and walks: all reflect the personality. Even the mode of dress may indicate the life style and therefore the stresses and strains that are put on the feet. Footwear can be the main contributory factor in foot problems of a local mechanical nature, and its observation is therefore particularly important.

Getting an initial general impression is vital and should not be hurried. Adequate time should be allowed for patients to state what is troubling them. Clues may be picked up to systemic disorders.

There is a wide range of shape, size, mobility and colour which constitutes normality in the feet. The criterion is simply that the feet should be such that they allow a reasonable range of activities to be undertaken, commensurate with a patient's age and general health, in a pain-free manner, and that they can be accommodated in readily available footwear. No obvious pathological process should be present.

Compare the feet for symmetry and general configuration. They can be viewed from medial, lateral, dorsal and posterior aspects, both on weight bearing and at rest. The plantar view is the most revealing of how the body weight is distributed. Observation of gait is important. Manipulation of joints at rest, to assess the range of movement, muscle power and alteration in temperature and sensation, assists in confirming visual impressions.

Look for asymmetry or swelling, and attempt to deduce the reason for it. If any oedema is present, the patient's history may indicate if it is due to recent physical trauma or has a systemic cause. Oedema may be physiological, due to prolonged standing on a hot day with delay in venous and lymphatic return. If it is accompanied by erythema, it could indicate inflammation of the underlying soft tissues; this may have arisen either by infection in the area, or aseptically as in tenosynovitis or muscle overuse. Soft tissue swelling could also indicate inflammation of bursae from pressure or friction over bony prominences, especially over the medial aspect of the first meta-tarsophalangeal (1st mtp) joint and the tendo Achilles area. Fatty tissue deposits may be found near the lateral malleoli. Bony prominences can indicate malalignment of bones and hence of joints, as when the first metatarsal (1st mt) head moves medially in hallux valgus, or—when located on the dorsum of the 1st mtp joint—osteophytic lipping in hallux rigidus; they are also found on the dorsum of the foot at the base of the 1st and 2nd mt and the cuneiform bones in tarsal osteo-arthritis.

For an accurate assessment of their colour, feet should be observed in daylight. Colour distribution and change in the foot when the leg is dependent or raised can indicate the efficiency of the arterial and venous circulation. Note any marked local change, such as cyanosis in a digit which may indicate local ischaemia even when the dorsalis pedis and posterior tibial pulses are palpable. Cyanosis occurs also on chilling. Pallor is normal in low ambient temperatures, but if prolonged under warm conditions it may indicate underlying disorders such as Raynaud's phenomenon. Colour changes occur in a variety of skin disorders. Particular attention should be paid to any locally pigmented areas of skin, especially if any change has occurred.

Alteration to the epidermis and underlying tissues occurs in skin disorders, and may range from vesicle formation in fungal infections, or pustules in psoriasis, to ulceration in diabetes. The normal texture of the skin varies from moist, elastic and warm in the young, to dryer, inelastic and cooler in the older individual. Increase in sweating occurs if the foot is kept in a warm atmosphere and particularly if occlusive footwear is worn; it will also occur when the person is under stress or in pain, or as a result of some metabolic disorder.[2] Hyperhidrosis encourages the spread of fungal infection, which is frequently encountered in the medial longitudinal arch area and between the digits where maceration and fissuring are found.

Look at the nails. In the young they are thinner, more flexible and translucent, becoming thicker, duller and less malleable with increasing age. Changes in shape, texture and colour can take

[1]The foot that shows nothing, yet when there appears to be nothing to see one can point out what there really is to see! A sort of informed looking which is the secret of observation, to know what to look for when there appears to be nothing to comment upon . . . 'eagle-eyed captain saves drowning sailors' . . . because the sea did not look empty and the inconsistencies were heads!

[2]Thyrotoxicosis, acromegaly, hyperhidrosis and hypoglycaemia all present with an increase in sweating.

place due to shoe pressure, which also allows fungal infection of the nail plate. Some typical nail changes accompany particular systemic disorders,[3] and the nail may reflect the quality of the arterial circulation to the limb, as may other of the skin appendages.

The feet are exposed to much physical stress and trauma in daily use and in recreation,[4] and any abnormality in weight bearing and joint alignment can give rise to mechanical inefficiency and deformity. There are common patterns of deformity, especially in shod societies.

Hallux valgus presents with splaying of the forefoot in the region of the metatarsal (MT) heads and disruption of the soft tissue involved. The lesser toes are crowded into a wedge shape and lose their function, often resulting in hammer and mallet toe deformity. The middle three mt heads are overloaded on the plantar surface and there is flattening of the medial longitudinal arch.

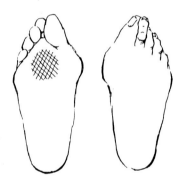

Valgus foot occurs when the tarsal area rolls medially, altering the pitch of the calcaneum and causing the forefoot to move away from the midline of the body. The medial longitudinal arch disappears. This is seen in the poorly controlled hypermobile foot and in feet which have been subjected to prolonged standing and overloading.

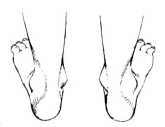

Pes cavus indicates an exaggerated medial longitudinal arch, and non-weight bearing on the lateral border; in mild cases the foot remains mobile with little retraction of the toes, and few mechanical problems arise.

[3]Clubbing, pitting, koilonychia, Beau's lines.
[4]Footballer's foot in the barefoot African, and the farmer in Nigeria with hookworm or the trauma of anaesthetic leprosy.

A typical **mobile cavus foot** has diffuse plantar callus under the 2nd, 3rd and 4th mt heads. A **rigid cavus foot** has more severe callus/corns (which may be very painful) under the 1st and 5th mt heads. It is associated with a central band of plantar fascia pulling the mt heads up. More severe cases, often accompanying neurological disorders, are associated with gross retraction of the toes and overloading of the 1st and 5th mt heads. Pressure lesions occur on these overloaded areas,[5] and there is a stiff ungainly gait.

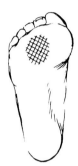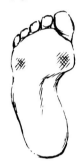

Hallux rigidus (66) implies limitation or absence of dorsiflexion at the first mt joint. In the acute condition the immobility is due to pain and effusion in the joint, caused by trauma—as with stubbing the great toe; in the chronic variety osteoarthritic changes occur, with osteophytic lipping on the dorsum preventing dorsiflexion. The gait is altered, the forefoot turning outward by external rotation at the hip.

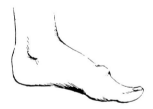

The best guide to the overloading of areas of the foot, and an indication of the way that the foot functions, is the colour, thickness and changes in the structure of the skin on the sole. The precise position of corns, callus, and even ulceration— and the relationship of these to underlying bony structures—is significant, as are skin creases caused by repetitive movements, and the quality and disposition of fibrofatty tissue.

Devices which measure pressure loading on different parts of the plantar surface are useful for static load estimation at a single second in time, but they cannot indicate the shearing stress in the tissues on movement when bearing body weight and wearing shoes.

[5]Producing the classic perforating ulcer in diabetes, tabes and leprosy.

3 The foot and the normal range

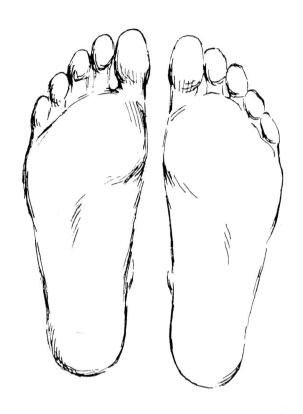

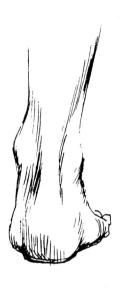

The shape of a normal foot

(i) **From the plantar aspect** with the foot at right angles to the leg, neither inverted nor everted, and at the eye level of the observer.

- Foot should be a mirror image of its pair.
- Size and position of the pulp (pads) of the toes indicate their position and functioning.
- Lateral border fairly straight with epidermal evidence of weight taken in this area.[6]
- Heel contour should suggest good fibrofatty padding, well attached to the underlying tissue.
- Medial border with moderate arching and skin creasing indicating mobility.
- Medial malleolus just visible. If placed more medially it would suggest a valgus foot on weight bearing.
- No undue splaying of the foot in the region of the mt heads.
- Surface should be free from corns, and callus present should be physiological and appear over the heel, lateral border, over the metatarsal head area and the pulp of the toes.

[6]Of skin thickening due to weight bearing.

(ii) **Posterior view**

- Tendo Achilles passes medially down the leg before being inserted into the calcaneum. The medial and lateral malleoli should be evenly placed on either side, although at different levels.

68–77 Examples of normal feet from a class of six-year-old children, identified by sex and ethnic origin.

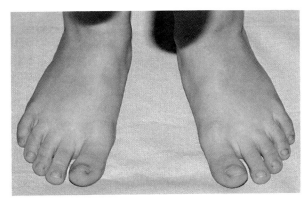

68

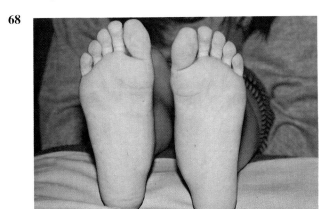

70

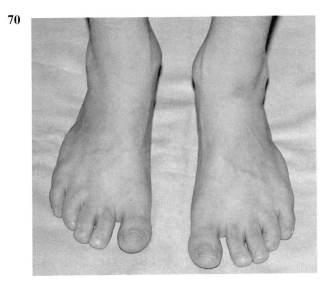

72

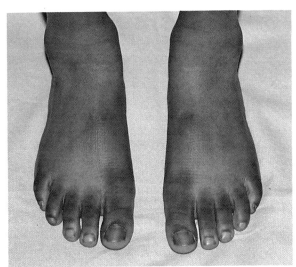

69

71

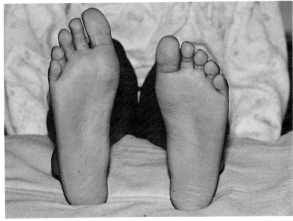

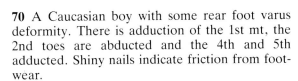

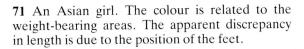

68 An Asian girl. The fullness on the medial border indicates some pronation which is present on weight bearing. The skin creases over the 1st metatarsophalangeal (MTP) joint are normal.

69 An Asian girl. Mild plano valgus feet, more marked on the left foot. Both big toes tend to hyperextend. An old injury to the right nail shows a growth arrest line.

70 A Caucasian boy with some rear foot varus deformity. There is adduction of the 1st mt, the 2nd toes are abducted and the 4th and 5th adducted. Shiny nails indicate friction from foot-wear.

71 An Asian girl. The colour is related to the weight-bearing areas. The apparent discrepancy in length is due to the position of the feet.

72 A West Indian boy with rotation and burrowing of the 5th toes; this often results in interdigital corns and callus if tight shoes are worn. The pigment distribution on the dorsum is normal.

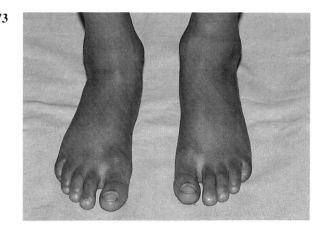

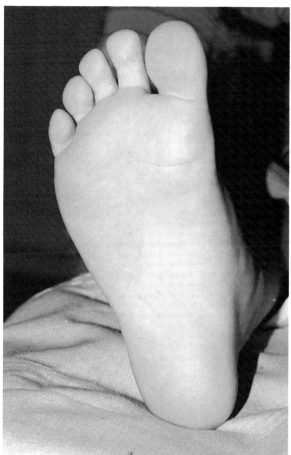

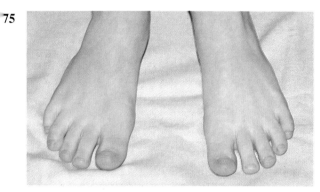

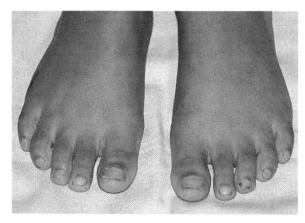

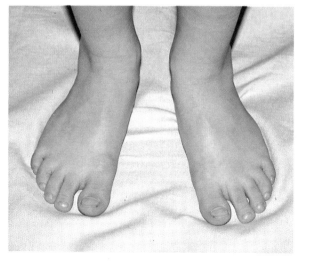

73 A West Indian boy with rotation and burrowing of the 5th toes. The shiny nails are the result of friction from footwear.

74 A Caucasian boy. Callus over the 5th mt head indicates that more weight is taken on the lateral forefoot.

75 A Caucasian girl with a tendency to pronate on both feet. There is hyperextension at the interphalangeal joints of big toes. Prominence of the tendon of extensor digitorum longus of the left foot is a temporary balancing mechanism.

76 An Asian boy with some adduction and rotation of the 4th and 5th toes.

77 A Caucasian boy with a plano valgus posture, which is common at this age and usually corrects itself without treatment.

78–104 The range of normal in different age groups.

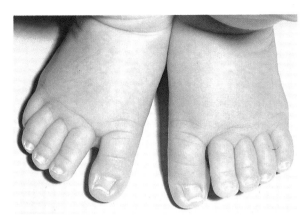

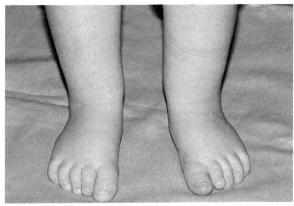

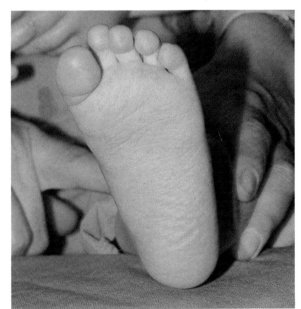

78 An infant of six months, with the involuted nails and bulging nail folds which are common at this age.

79 and 80 A girl aged nine months. The normal flat appearance of the medial longitudinal arch seen in **79** is due to fatty tissue in the sole. There is functional clawing of the toes on standing. The plantar aspect is shown in **80**.

81 A girl aged one year who is not yet walking, but who shows lesser toe moulding from wearing tight all-in-one stretch garments. No family history of curly toes.

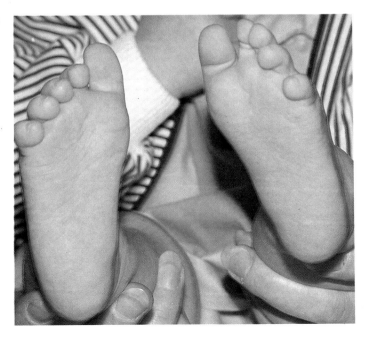

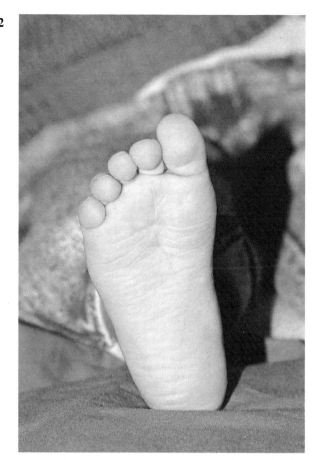

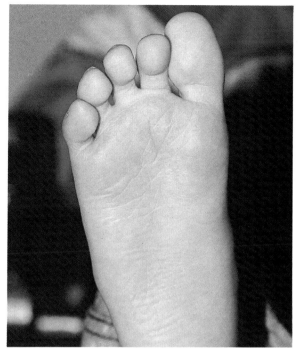

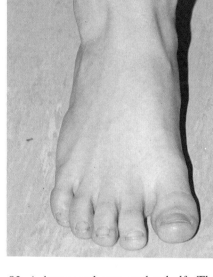

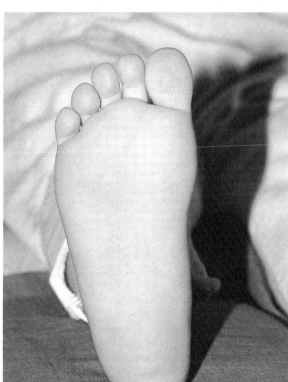

82 A boy aged two and a half. The visible nail plates indicate increased flexion of the lesser toes. The skin creases are normal.

83 A girl aged four years. Good position of all toes.

84 and 85 A boy aged eight. There is some pinching of the plantar fibrofatty pad near the base of the toes. The base of the 5th mt is prominent on the lateral border. There is coarseness of the skin on the plantar surface. The boy was accompanied by his mother, who has hyperkeratosis of the palms and soles.

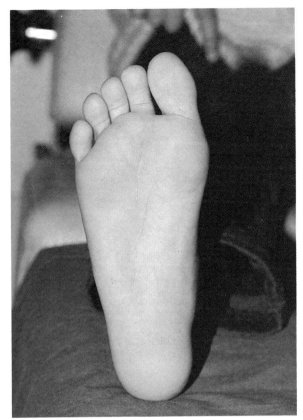

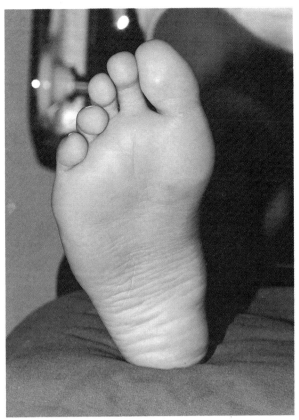

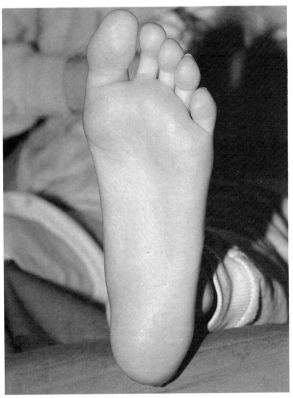

86 A boy from Trinidad aged nine. The contours and colour changes show the weight-bearing areas.

87 A Turkish boy aged 12. He is a keen runner. The position of the foot and the skin creases at rest indicate a mobile foot. More weight is taken on the lateral border and over the lateral three mt heads. There is increased plantar flexion of the 4th and 5th toes.

88 A girl of 13 years. A long slim foot shows some elevation of the 1st and 2nd mt. The heel is narrow and shoe fitting may be a problem as she gets older.

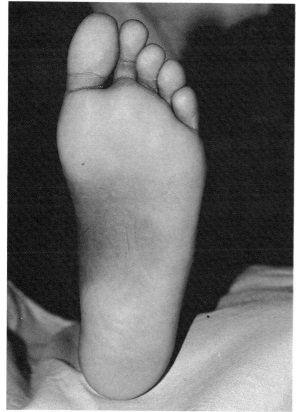

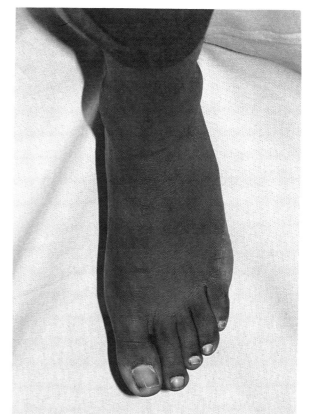

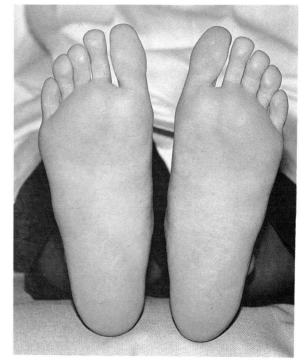

89 and 90 A West Indian boy of 14 with a long second toe. The skin creases and texture under the medial longitudinal arch indicate the firm tethering of the subcutaneous tissue.

91 A female student aged 20 with long slim feet, the left one slightly narrower. There is a small verruca on the pulp of the left big toe.

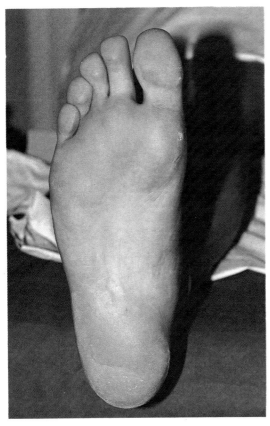

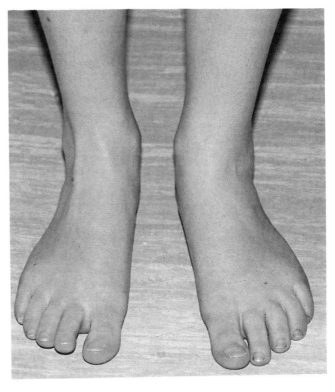

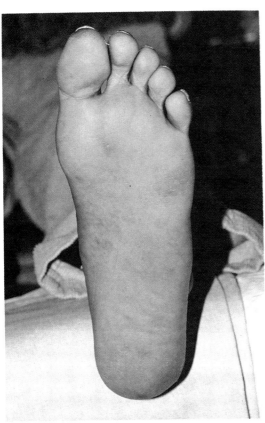

92 A 20-year-old woman with a highly arched foot and tight plantar fascia. There is callus on the medial border from nipping between the upper and sole of her shoe, and white talcum powder is present.

93 A 21-year-old woman with some inrolling of the left foot. The tendons of extensor digitorum longus and tibialis anterior are tense on the right foot as she balances.

94 A West Indian male of 22 years. Callus over 2nd and 5th mt heads shows the site of extra loading. The pigmentation is normal.

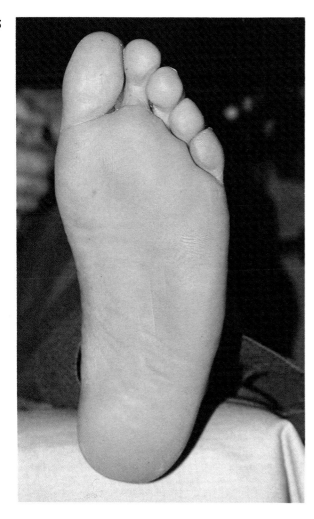

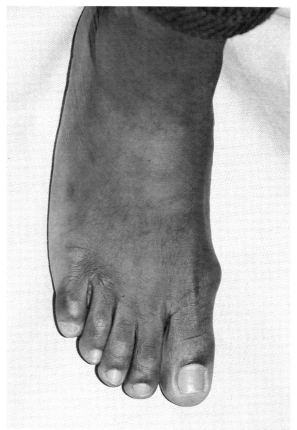

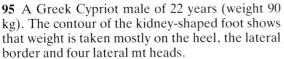

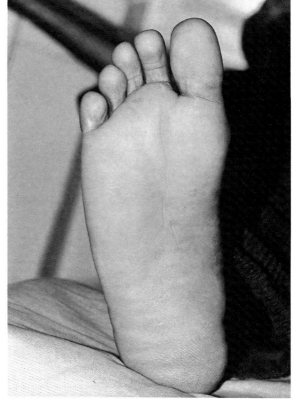

95 A Greek Cypriot male of 22 years (weight 90 kg). The contour of the kidney-shaped foot shows that weight is taken mostly on the heel, the lateral border and four lateral mt heads.

96 and 97 A Nigerian male aged 23. There is a small bony prominence on the medial border of the 1st mt head (**96**). There is a full range of movement at the joint, although skin creases on the dorsum of the big toe suggest rotation on walking. The small seed corns on the plantar surface (**97**) near the heel are often found in dry skins.

98

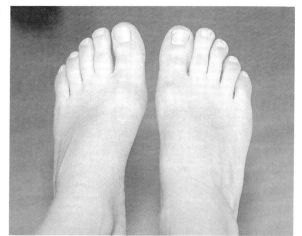

98 A woman aged 31. The nails are thin, and there are wide nail folds on the big toes, and there is a tendency to hyperextension at the inter-phalangeal joints. The direction of longitudinal ridges on the nails shows they are pushed laterally by footwear. Shoe pressure is also apparent at the medial side of the free edge of the nails.

99

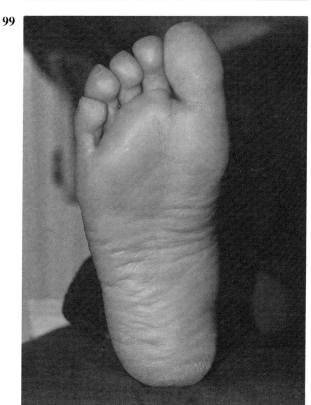

10●

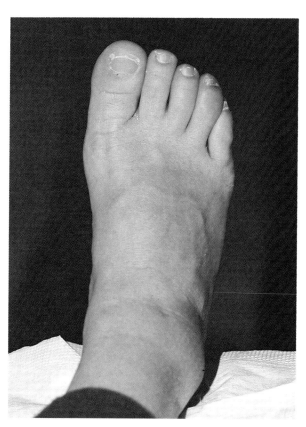

99 and 100 A Chinese woman aged 50 years. The long 4th toe has been pushed back into line by footwear, resulting in pressure on the distal phalanx (**99**). The 5th toe burrows under the 4th. The nails have been cut too short (**100**), allowing the soft tissue to roll over the free edge and causing discomfort. There is a pad of fatty tissue near the right lateral malleolus, a common finding in older women.

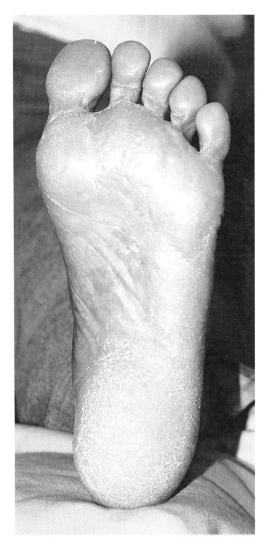

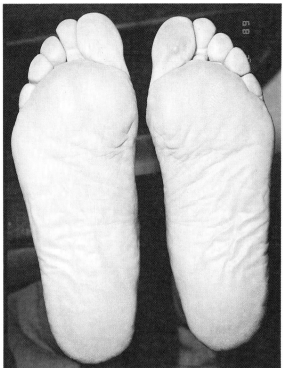

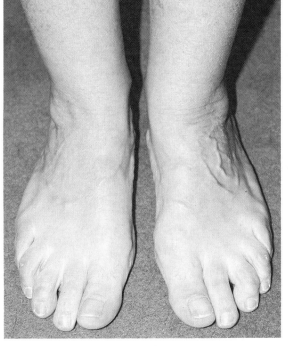

101 An Asian man of 58 years. There is typical dry texture and tethering of the skin and subcutaneous tissue. The position of the toes at rest is good, but the ridge of callus near the base of the 4th toe shows how the 5th toe burrows when shoes are worn. The seed corns near the heel are common in dry skin. The superficial callus over the lateral mt heads has been pared away.

102–103 A woman aged 65. At rest, mild plano valgus feet with slight hallux valgus (**102**). Dilated superficial veins are apparent on the dorsum. The reduced elasticity of the ageing skin is shown by skin folds on the plantar surface (**102**). A small fibroma is evident on the pulp of left great toe.

In activity, the foot arches and the plano valgus posture disappears.

4 Footwear

Any covering on the feet can affect foot function, especially if it is of a restrictive nature. The advent of stretch hosiery adds to the problem. With the demands of fashion and the personal preference of most women, if foot health is to be maintained into later years some form of compromise is needed. To wear two different types of shoe—one more 'sensible' for use when standing and walking (and for any sporting activity not requiring specialist footwear), and the other for more formal occasions—is preferable to wearing a compromise most of the time.[1]

General points in shoe fitting

- Shoe should be long enough to accommodate the foot on standing (when it tends to lengthen) and care should be taken to avoid stretch hose pulling back the toes.

4A

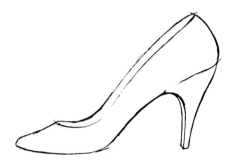

- Toe box of the shoe must be deep enough to accommodate the depth of the toes and the forepart round enough to accommodate all of the toes, especially in a broad foot.
- If the shoe is fitted as above there must be some means of holding the shoe on to the foot if the heel is not to leave the shoe on heel lift in walking! Therefore, all slip-on shoes, including closed-in slippers, must be too short if the shoe is to stay on the foot in walking. Lacing, which is adjustable, is best for sensible shoe wear, but it must be functional and not merely decorative.
- Heel should be low enough to allow the body weight to be distributed evenly over the sole

[1]Extremes are better than the middle path!

(hind- to forefoot). The surface area of the heel must be large enough to give stability and to avoid stress at the ankle joint. Lower heels prevent shortening of the posterior calf group of muscles.

If higher heels are worn, the more easily moulded forefoot is deformed.

104B

- Material of the sole should be flexible, waterproof, durable, and have insulating properties (cushioning and temperature).
- If woven fabric (warp and weft) is used, whether for lining or outer material in the upper, it can give rise to pressure lésions on prominent joints—unlined, leather-lined or jersey fabric lining is preferred.
- In cold weather, when lined boots or shoes or extra warm hose are used, allowance must be made in the size of the footwear.

Let firm well hammered soles protect thy feet
Thro' freezing snows and rains and soaking sleet.
Should the big last extend the shoe too wide
Each stone will wrench the unwary step aside:
The sudden turn may stretch the swelling vein
The cracking joint unhinge, or ankle sprain,
And when too short the modish shoes are worn
You'll judge the seasons by your shooting corn.

John Gay (1685–1732), English poet and dramatist, in *Trivia or the art of walking the streets of London*, Book 1, 33.

5 The shoe-moulded foot: functionally normal

Like the hands, the shape of the feet may not be an accurate guide to comfort and function, often reflecting the lifestyle and footwear of the individual's formative younger years, decades earlier.

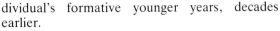

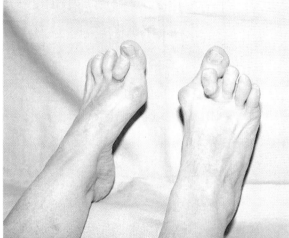

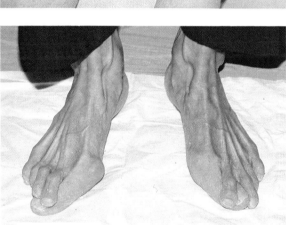

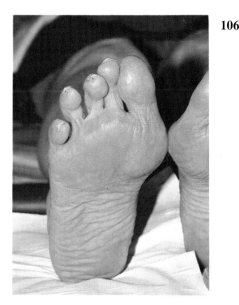

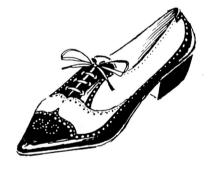

105–117 Elderly feet, male and female, though usually misshapen by footwear in youth, now cause few or no problems when adequately shod. The people featured here are all active individuals.

105 A woman aged 67 years with **bilateral hallux valgus.** There is dorsal displacement and adduction of the 2nd toes with soft tissue thickening over the proximal interphalangeal joints from shoe rub. The right second metatarsophalangeal (2nd mtp) joint is dislocated and the increased width of the forefoot is due to the first metatarsal (1st mt) moving medially.

106 Hallux valgus—the mobile foot of a 72-year-old woman. There are corns on the apices of the 3rd and 4th toes, and the shape of toe-flexure folds indicates how the forefoot is moulded by the court shoes she still wears.

107 A 74-year-old man with **bilateral hallux valgus** with dorsal displacement, adduction of both 2nd toes and the 3rd on the right foot. In lean feet the tendons of tibialis anterior, extensor hallucis longus and extensor digitorum longus are obvious. He worked in the fashion trade for many years, wearing pointed-toed shoes (**diagram**).

39

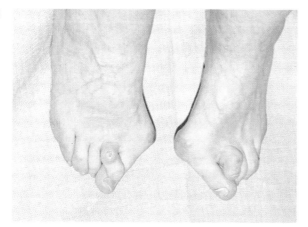

108–110 This 75-year-old woman wore high-heeled court shoes for many years. She has **bilateral hallux valgus** with rotation of the big toes, and shoe pressure has caused a thickening of the left great toe nail. The 2nd toes are dorsally displaced, the right adducted with corn and callus over the proximal interphalangeal joints. On standing (**109**), there is tension in the tendons of tibialis anterior, extensor digitorum longus and extensor hallucis longus, resulting from an attempt to stabilise the foot: this is absent when the feet are at rest (**108**). The trapping of the 2nd toes transfers pressure from the dorsum on to the mt heads (**110**).

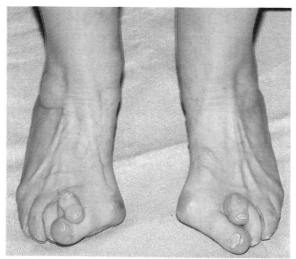

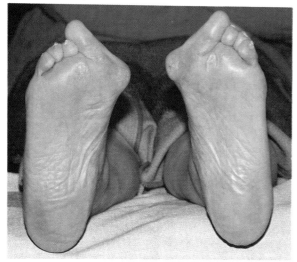

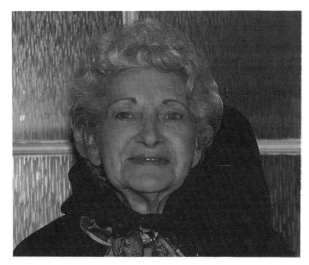

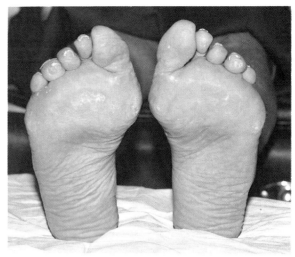

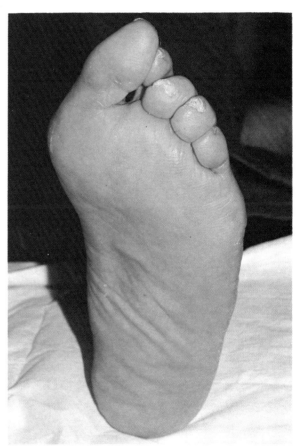

111 and 112 An 81-year-old former fashion model, who still enjoys wearing high-heeled court shoes, is pictured in **111**. Moderate bilateral hallux valgus and the clawing of the lesser toes causes corns on the apices of the fourth toes (**112**). The feet are mobile. The fibrofatty padding over the mt heads has moved distally, leaving the weight-bearing areas uncushioned and tied down to the underlying tissue—hence the flattened appearance with overlying callus.

113 A man aged 81 years—a mobile foot with good fibrofatty padding with hallux valgus and dorsal displacement of the second toe but the forefoot has avoided the usual marked overloading of the second metatarsal head on the plantar surface. The increase in plantar flexion of the third and fourth toes has caused thickening of the nails.

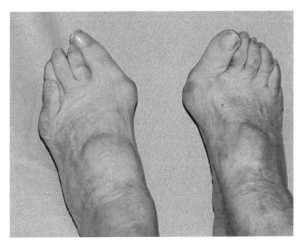

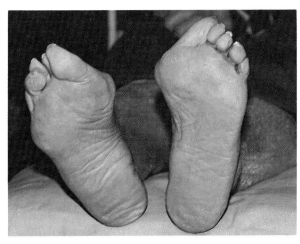

114 and 115 A woman of 82 years, presenting with **bilateral hallux valgus** and crowding of the lesser toes adopting a differing position in each foot (**114**). This is often associated with original foot length discrepancy. In the left foot the 1st mt head has moved medially and all the toes have resisted pressure from the big toe. In the right foot the 2nd toe has moved dorsally, and the 4th toe burrows under the third producing a corn where the rotation causes pressure (**115**). The 5th toe is adducted. There is some tarsal arthritis with soft tissue swelling on the dorsum.

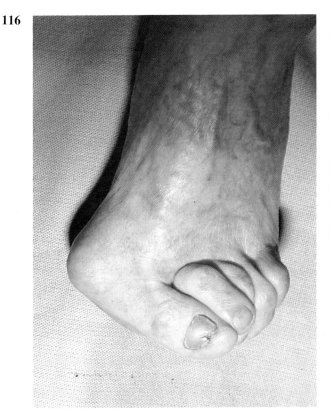

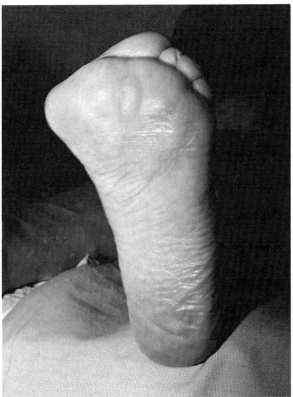

116 and 117 The gross hallux valgus, seen in a cheerful and fit 92-year-old woman who worked full time as a laboratory assistant until 79 years of age. She remains active, and comfortable, in mass-produced footwear.

6 The painful foot due to local mechanical problems

Most problems of painful feet are found in the easily moulded forefoot, and many cases reflect the wearing of inadequate footwear. Malalignment of joints leads to mechanical disadvantage in weight bearing and mobility. The extra stress on the tissues that results causes painful recurring problems, with the mechanical distortions becoming irreversible even if suitable shoes are worn.

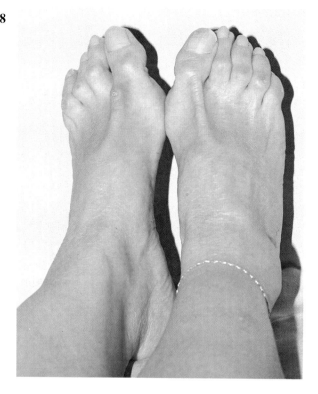

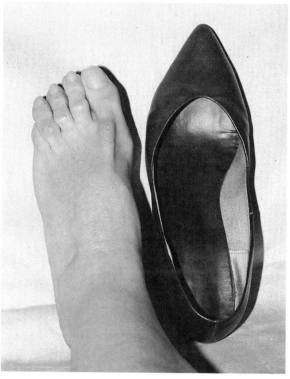

118 and 119 Mild hallux valgus of both feet with dorsiflexion at the metatarsophalangeal (MTP) joints and plantar flexion at the interphalangeal joints. Both extensor hallucis longus tendons are very tight with dorsal bowstringing. There is a deep painful fibrous corn over the left tendon where the rim of the court shoe opening rubs. It is the site of an old sinus tracking down to the tendon sheath.

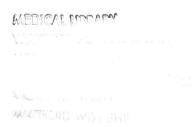

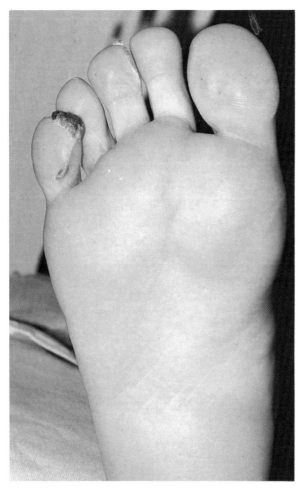

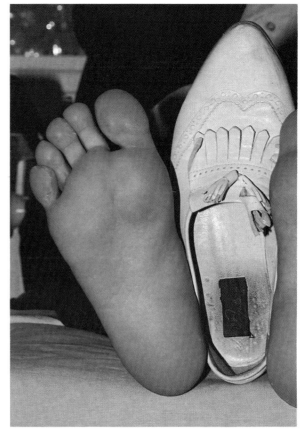

120 and 121 The broad forefoot of a Turkish waiter aged 23 years (**120**). Squeezing the foot into pointed-toe shoes (**121**) has resulted in burrowing of the 5th toe under the 4th toe. The great toe has resisted valgus positioning. A painful ridge of callus has formed, discoloured by bleeding into the callus. The side of the middle toe also has callus from pressure.

122

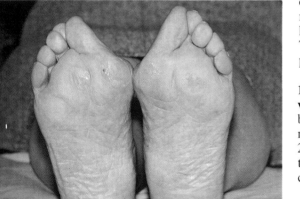

122 A woman of 70 years with **bilateral hallux valgus** and rotation of the toes. The 2nd toes have been displaced dorsally with typical triangular moulding of the pulps. Overloading of the 1st and 2nd metatarsal (MT) heads of the right foot and the 3rd of the left foot has resulted in painful callus.

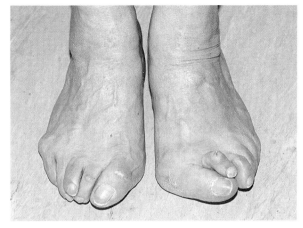

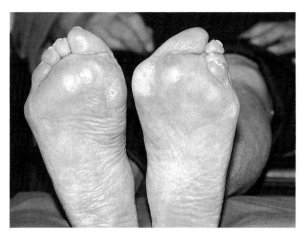

123 and 124 Gross bilateral hallux valgus in a woman of 80 years. In the left foot (**123**) the 2nd toe is dorsally dislocated and abducted at the mtp joint with a painful corn over the proximal interphalangeal (IP) joint from shoe rub. The 3rd toe has also moved laterally and overlies the 4th and 5th toes. Overloading of the 2nd MT head has resulted in painful plantar callus (**124**). In the right foot (**123**) the 3rd toe has moved dorsally and the big toe is plantar-flexed at the IP joint. There is plantar overloading on the 2nd and 3rd MT heads (**124**).

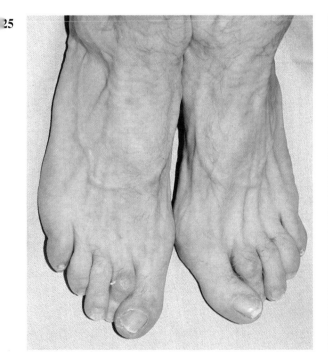

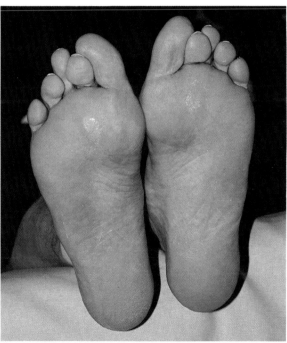

125 and 126 Bilateral hallux valgus, more marked at the IP joints, in a man of 62 years (**125**). The 2nd toes have adapted to the displacement by fixed plantar flexion at the proximal IP joints (hammer toes) with painful pressure lesions on the dorsum. The plantar view (**126**) shows the typical overloading of the 2nd MT heads. In these lean feet the tendons and the superficial veins are easily identified.

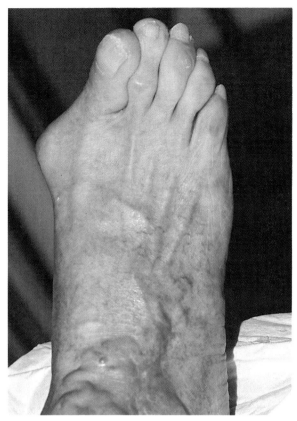

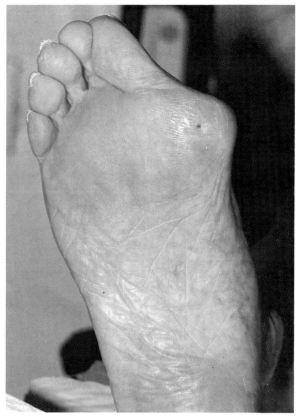

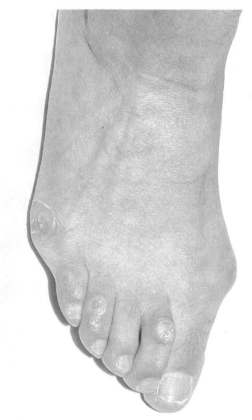

127 and 128 Hallux valgus with rotation of the toe (**127**). The 2nd toe has resisted displacement, the position of the hallux having been achieved by adduction of the 1st MT. There is only moderate callus from overload of the 1st MT head (**128**). Dilated superficial veins and an area of atrophie blanche[1] near the lateral malleolus are visible over the leg and dorsum of the foot.

129 Hallux valgus, with splaying in the region of the MT heads by increased angulation between 1:2 and 4:5 MT, has resulted in a painful callosity over the lateral border of the foot. The 2nd toe is hammered and pressure lesions occur on it and the 4th and 5th toes.

[1]Atrophie blanche: obliteration of capillaries in the upper dermis, causing sclerosis. Residual vessels are attenuated and liable to thrombosis and consequent ulceration. Seen with gravitational stasis and venous obstruction, as well as with many vasculitides.

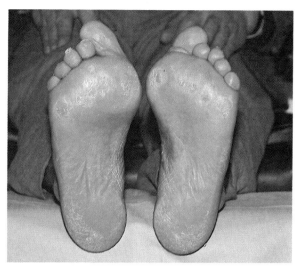

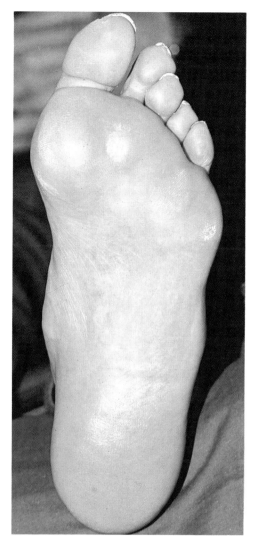

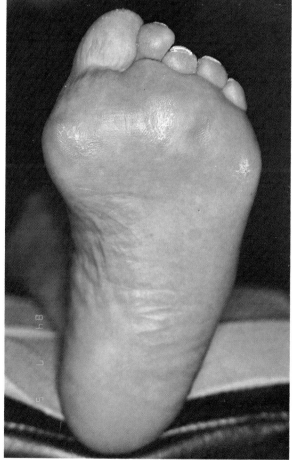

130 A man of 56 years, a heavy smoker, with a fairly **mobile cavus foot**. There is moderate hallux valgus and adduction of the 5th toe. The fibro-fatty tissue over the forefoot has moved distally, resulting in painful callus on the 2nd, 1st and 5th MT heads. The subcutaneous tissue under the medial longitudinal arch is firmly tethered.

131 Bilateral cavus feet in an elderly man. The plantar fascia is tight. All lesser toes are retracted and the valgus position of the big toe on the right foot traps the 2nd into plantar flexion, with plantar callus on the apex of the toe and plantar pad. The fibro-fatty tissue over the MT head has moved distally, resulting in callus formation over the MT head. The dusky appearance of the feet is due to peripheral ischaemia.

132 A man aged 58 years with **mobile cavus feet** and retraction of the toes. There is typical displacement of the fibro-fatty pad distally, leaving weight-bearing areas dimpled with painful callus over the 1st, 2nd and 5th MT heads.

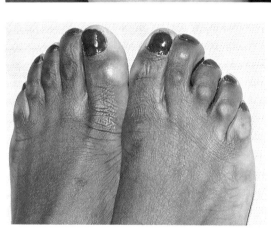

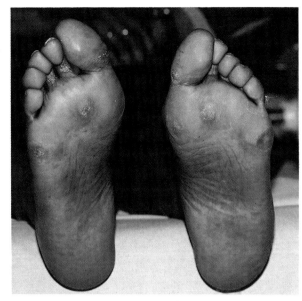

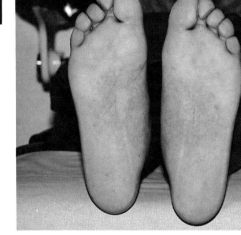

133 A man aged 61 years with a congenital low-arched **mobile foot** and short 4th and 5th toes. Less weight is taken on the 1st mt head, and the ridge of callus near the 1st interdigital cleft indicates a pivotal movement on walking.

134 A West Indian woman of 27 years with early **bilateral hallux valgus**. There is tethering of the tissues under the medial longitudinal arch which lowers considerably on standing. The wearing of plastic, inelastic occlusive thin-soled shoes has caused scaling in the flexor surfaces of the toes. There is thick painful callus on the big toes and over the 2nd and 5th MT heads (some callus has been removed from the left 5th area).

135 and 136 A West Indian woman of 25 years with early moulding of the feet from wearing high-heeled court shoes (**135**). The big toe is in valgus at the IP joint with soft tissue thickening on the dorsum. All lesser toes show similar thickening over the proximal IP joints. The plantar view (**136**) reveals triangular moulding of the pulp of the 2nd toes as they are pushed dorsally. The outline of the insole of the short shoe can be seen as a pale line around the heel and along the medial and lateral borders.

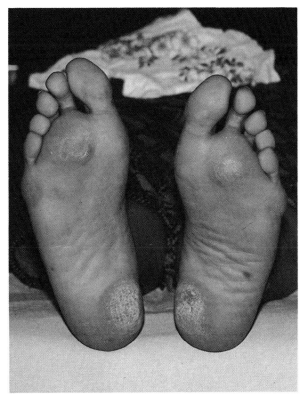

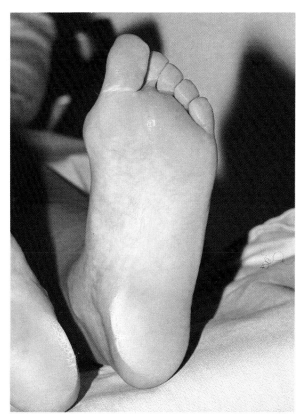

137 A Greek Cypriot woman of 43 years with **mobile feet**. Tight footwear has caused crowding of the toes to the shape of the shoe. Poor toe function has increased the load on the 2nd MT head with a painful callus. Inrolling of the heels on weight bearing has produced similar callus on the medial border.

138 A woman aged 44 years with painful **plantar callus** over the 2nd MT head where the toe is moving dorsally. The position of similar callus over the heels indicates the short high-heeled shoes worn. The patient is a heavy smoker.

139 An Asian man of 56 years with typical dry tethered skin and painful plantar corns. In the forefoot the corns are associated with poor toe function; those near the heels are old injuries resulting from walking barefoot in Bangladesh. Some callus has been removed from the corns.

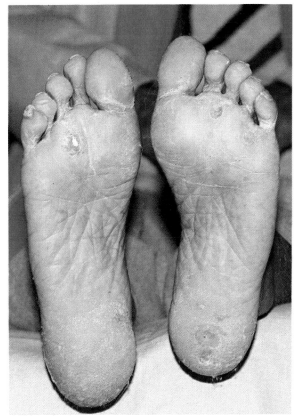

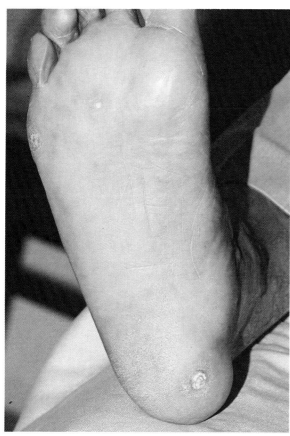
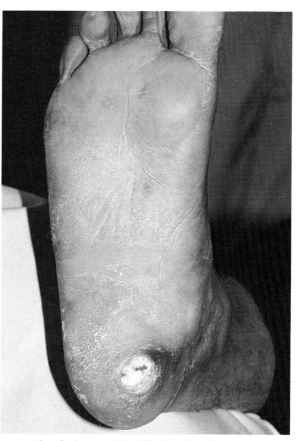

140 and 141 A Bangladeshi man of 58 years with **a painful corn** over the medial aspect of the heel (**140**) associated with an old injury acquired while working barefoot in his youth. There are corns over the 3rd and 5th MT heads. The pain was treated by cushioning, but six months later squamous cell carcinoma was revealed (**141**).

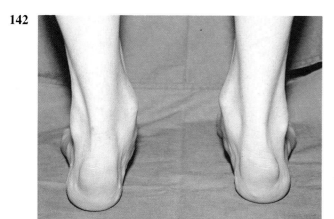
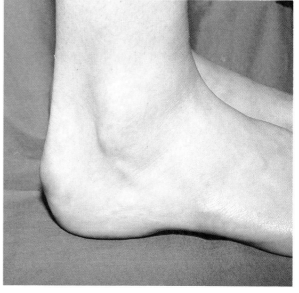

142 and 143 A young woman with **rear foot varus and heel bumps** (**143**). On weight bearing the feet pronate excessively to allow the inverted foot to become plantigrade.

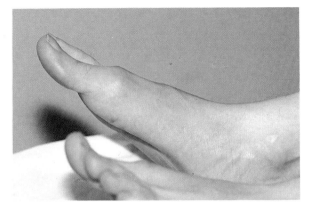

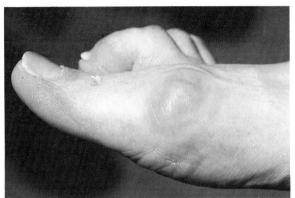

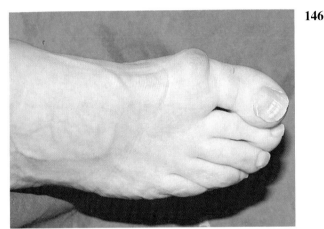

144 A young woman with **hallux flexus** in a poorly controlled foot. In an attempt to stabilise the distal part of the medial longitudinal arch the big toe is plantar-flexed at the MTP joint and hyperextended at the IP joint, a mechanism to compensate for an inverted heel or forefoot. Later changes often involve osteoarthritis at the MTP joint with bony lipping preventing dorsiflexion. Painful callus develops on the proximal part of the pulp of the big toe.

145 Hallux rigidus with an inability to dorsiflex at the 1st MTP joint due to arthritic changes within the joint and bony lipping on the dorso medial aspect. The colour change and skin crease on the big toe indicate stress on soft tissues as the IP joint attempts passive compensatory movement.

146 Hallux rigidus associated with violent stubbing of the toe years ago. There is a large exostosis on the medial aspect of the joint, and the thinned overlying tissue is exposed to shoe pressure and develops chilblains in cold weather.

147 A young woman with **a large fibrosed bursa** under the 1st MTP joint because of a very mobile and plantar-flexed 1st ray, with excessive movement reflected in the position of the skin creases under the arch.

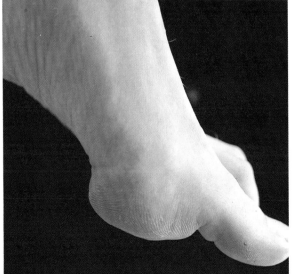

148

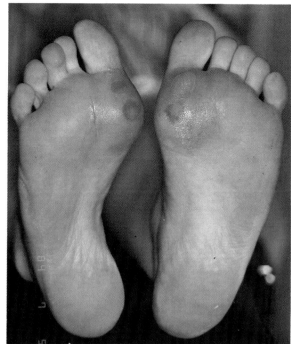

14

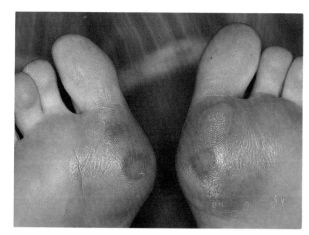

150

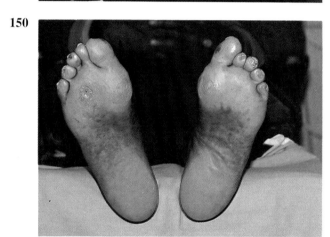

15

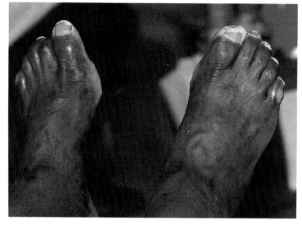

152

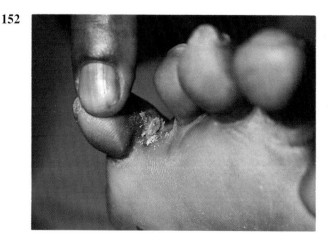

148 and 149 Cavus feet with tight plantar fascia, in a young woman squash player. Excessive rotational stress over the 1st MTP joint during play has produced blisters and bruising.

150 and 151 A West Indian road-sweeper aged 55 years. Fixed flexural deformity of all the toes (clawing) is associated with wearing short shoes. There are painful corns on the apices of most toes and the medial aspect of the big toes, with occasional ulceration—especially in cold weather. Painful callosities are seen over the 1st MT heads and the 3rd MT head on the right foot. The soft tissue is tightly tethered over the sole. Varicose veins on the dorsum are aggravated by prolonged standing at work.

152 A Jamaican man of 50 years with **a typical interdigital corn** in the 4th cleft made worse by a congenitally short 4th toe.

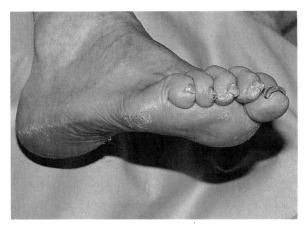

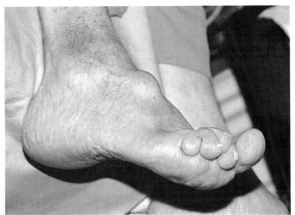

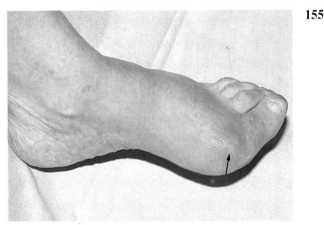

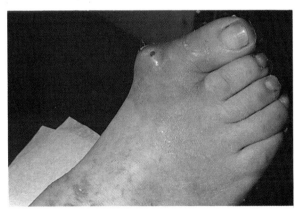

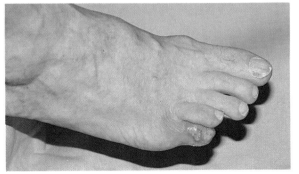

153 A gardener of 60 years whose feet are exposed to cold damp conditions for long periods. He has thickened **plantar-flexed nails and corns** on the apices of the 2nd and 3rd toes. There is some callus over the 5th MT head.

154 A man of 79 years with **a ganglion on the dorsum**. There is dorsal displacement of the 3rd toe and an apical corn from plantar flexion on the 4th with callus overlying the 3rd and 4th MT heads. There is a superficial resemblance to rheumatoid deformity.

155 A woman aged 79 years with **an infected oedematous bursa** over the 1st MTP joint. There is a small sinus just visible which is plugged with exudate. The big toe is adducted and rotated, and the nail has been damaged by shoe pressure.

156 An elderly woman with **an infected bursa and cyanosis** from chilling over the medial aspect of the 1st MTP joint. There is an exostosis but only moderate valgus position of the toe.

157 A man of 67 years with inflammation and ulceration on the 5th toe from self-treatment, with a proprietary cream, for a corn. The 4th toe is congenitally short. There is longitudinal separation of the nail from its bed (onycholysis), with characteristic discolouration suggestive of fungal infection.

158

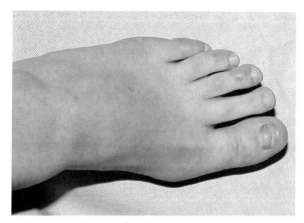

159

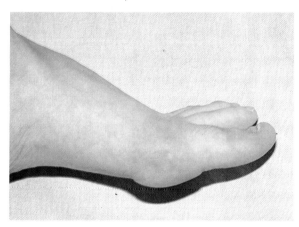

158 and 159 A young woman wore tight ski boots on a recent holiday, causing damage and shedding of the big toe nail (**158**). There are pressure lesions from footwear on the 3rd and 4th toes. The lateral view (**159**) shows bursal swelling under the 1st MT head from excessive movement.

160

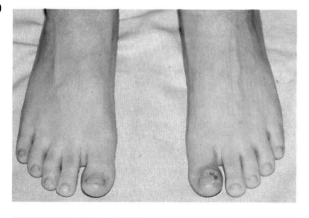

160 A six-year-old boy with an **ingrowing toe nail** and inflammation of the left big toe. The repeated rotational movement of a thin nail on the lateral sulcus in a young moist foot can result in infection and hypergranulation tissue. Short shoes and poor nail cutting are contributory factors.

161

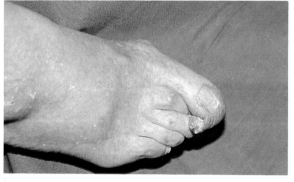

161 A woman aged 77 years with **a long thickened deformed great toe nail** which has pressed upon, but has not yet ulcerated, the 3rd toe. The 2nd toe is plantar-flexed from the valgus position of distal phalanx of the big toe. The oedema on the dorsum is limited distally by the edge of the shoe.

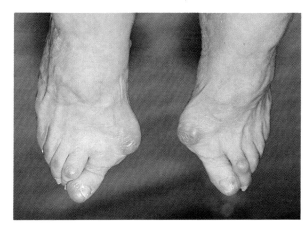

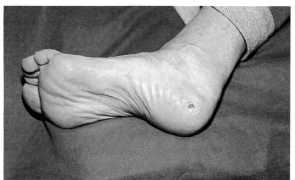

162 A woman of 74 years with **fungal infection** of the left big toe nail. She has **hallux valgus** of both feet with rotation of the toes and increased angulation between the 1st and 2nd MT. There are bursae from pressure and friction over the medial aspects of both 1st MT heads and the proximal IP joints of the 2nd toes.

163 A woman of 60 years with the **sequelae of a pressure sore** on the heel, after coma from drug overdose 20 years earlier. Healing resulted in much fibrous scar formation and a persistent painful corn with haemorrhagic breakdown in the centre.

164 and 165 A 28-year-old man who, as a result of a road accident, suffered a fracture and the loss of soft tissue, necessitating a skin graft on the medial aspect of the foot (**164**). There is an inability to dorsiflex the big toe, and an ulcer under the joint. Healing is apparent in **165**, with contraction of fibrous tissue and the small ulcer persisting. The inability to dorsiflex the big toe, together with the loss of soft tissue under the joint, will result in permanent problems of tissue breakdown unless the gait is altered to take the load on to the lateral forefoot.

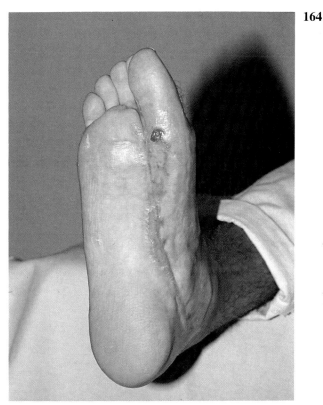

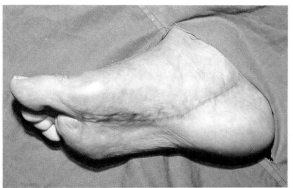

166

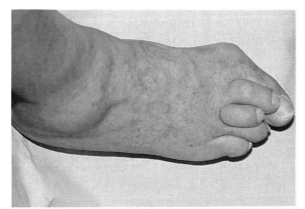

166 and 167 A man aged 75 years showing **gross hallux valgus**, with dorsal displacement of the 2nd and 3rd toes, following an accident involving MT fractures (**166**). Painful callus from overloading of the 3rd MT can be seen on the plantar surface (**167**). The left foot is normal.

167

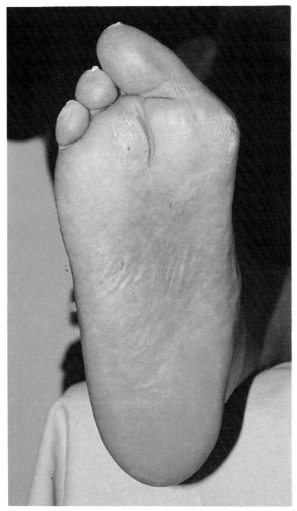

Minor congenital foot abnormalities which may lead to problems in later life

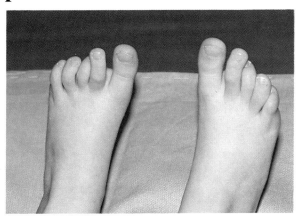

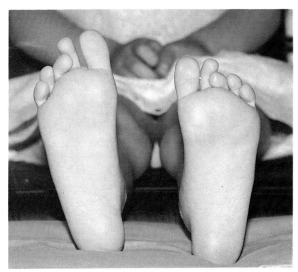

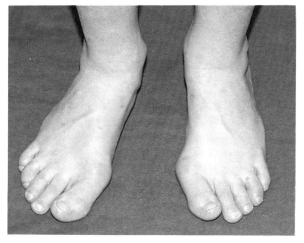

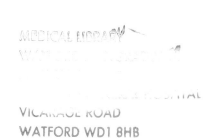

168 and 169 Congenital curly 3rd toes which burrow under the 2nd toe, in a girl aged six years. There is some adduction of the 1st MT. Her father has similar feet.

170 Early **hallux valgus** in a seven-year-old girl. The feet are pronated and there is medial rotation of the great toes indicating that the condition may deteriorate. The 1st ray is short. She has always worn well-fitting shoes. Her mother has similar feet.

171 Congenital burrowing of the 3rd toe, in a girl aged seven years. The condition is *not* present in the other foot. Footwear has always been adequate, and there is no family history of a similar deformity.

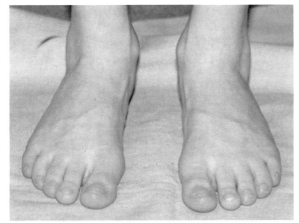

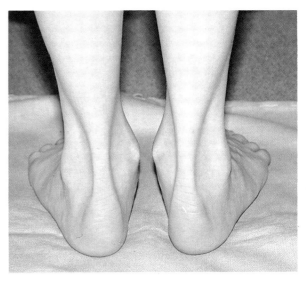

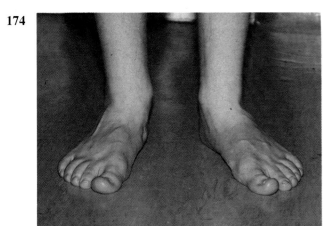

172 Pronated valgus feet in a girl aged 11 years.

173 Prominent **medial malleoli** with marks on apices where they rub against each other in walking. The subject has always worn suitable footwear; her father has similar feet.

174 and 175 Plano valgus feet in a boy aged 14 years (**174**). Father and grandfather have similarly shaped feet. Poor general posture and muscle tone are apparent. The boy dislikes physical exercise (but is good at mathematics!). There are heel bumps (**175**) from shoe rub over tendo Achilles.

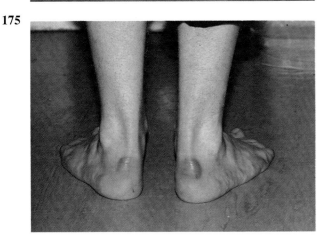

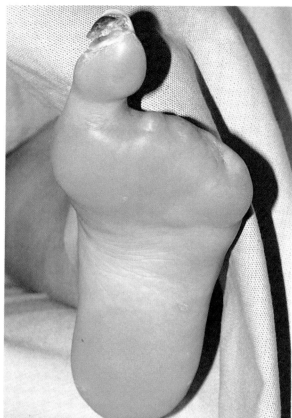

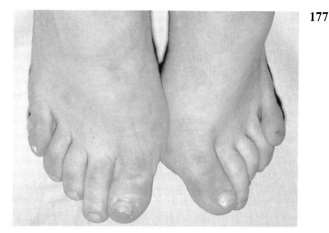

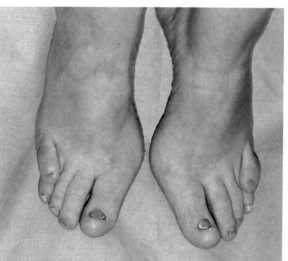

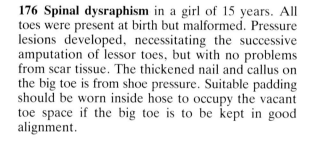

176 Spinal dysraphism in a girl of 15 years. All toes were present at birth but malformed. Pressure lesions developed, necessitating the successive amputation of lessor toes, but with no problems from scar tissue. The thickened nail and callus on the big toe is from shoe pressure. Suitable padding should be worn inside hose to occupy the vacant toe space if the big toe is to be kept in good alignment.

177 Poor toe configuration and function in a young girl. Early hallux valgus is present, with adduction of the 5th toes and high medial longitudinal arches, aggravated by poor footwear. Attempts to relieve pressure on the great toe nails have resulted in cutting them too short.

178 Highly arched feet with congenitally adducted 5th toes, in a woman of 55 years. Dystrophy of all nails and with red varnish.

179 Pes cavus and tight plantar fascia, in a girl of 16 years with a small heel area and a broad forefoot. No obvious neurological problem found. There is early callus over MT heads. No family history of a similar condition.

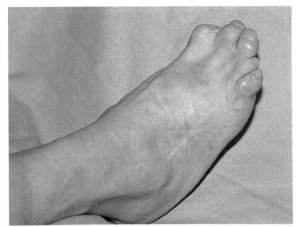

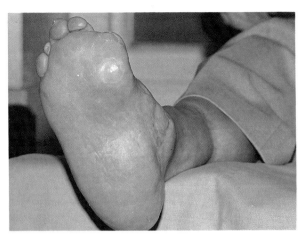

182

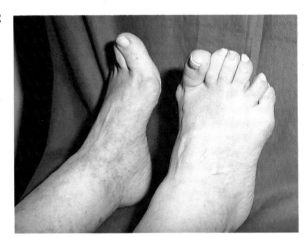

180 and 181 Congenital amniotic bands of the leg and foot (180) associated with deformities of the toes, in a 65-year-old man. Early surgery was necessary to achieve a plantigrade stable foot. There is callus on the 1st MT head, the base of the big toe space and the dorsum of the 5th toe (**181**). The deformities have not affected mobility.

182 Supernumerary toes on both feet; bifurcation of the 5th MT shaft. The subject had rudimentary tags on the lateral border of the hands removed surgically. She wears mass-produced wide shoes and has well-functioning feet.

183 Syndactyly of both feet with shiny nails from shoe rub—similar webbing of the hands was corrected surgically. No family history available.

183

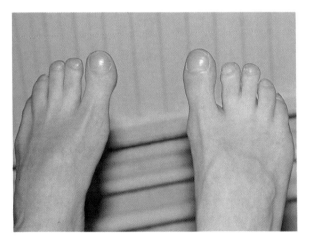

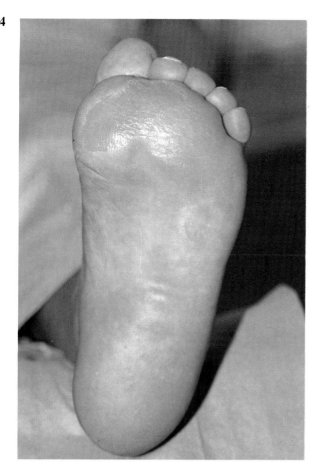

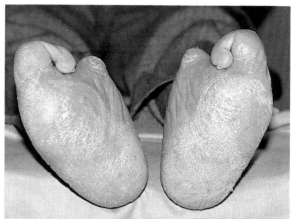

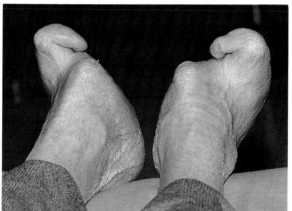

184 Mobile pes cavus, but limited dorsiflexion at the ankle joint and retracted toes, in a 53-year-old man. No spinal dysraphism. Callus over the 1st, 2nd and 3rd MT heads has been recently removed. Familial history of cavus feet.

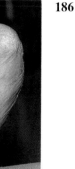

185–187 Lobster claw feet in a man of 76 years. In recent years a small area of callus has developed on the plantar surface of the right foot. He needs help cutting the single nail on each foot, his hands being similarly affected. He worked full time as a clerk and storekeeper from the age of 15 up to 65 years, maintaining his independence. He buys mass-produced shoes. His father, sister and niece share the same condition.

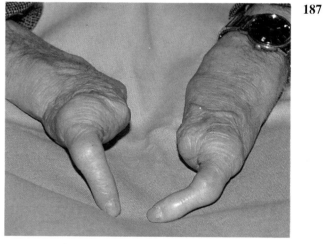

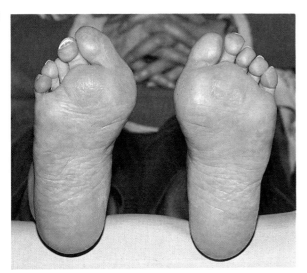

188 Congenitally short 3rd and 4th mt of the right foot and extra loading over the 2nd MT head. The 2nd toe is plantar-flexed. There is mottling from chilling on both feet in this 75-year-old woman.

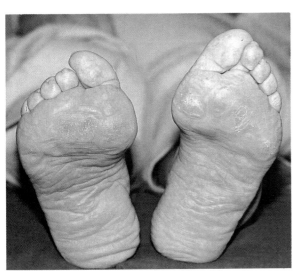

189 A congenital mobile cavus foot in a man of 60 years. The right is the more affected, with retracted toes. There is excessive movement in the soft tissues over the MT heads, with the formation of callus.

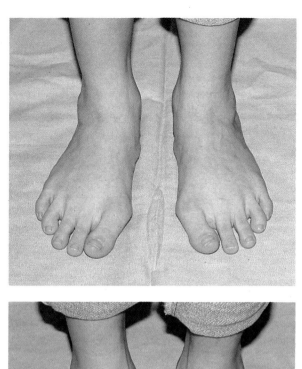

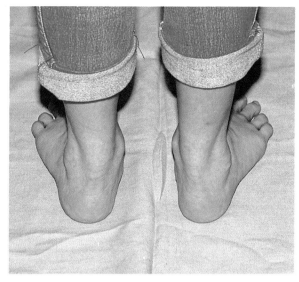

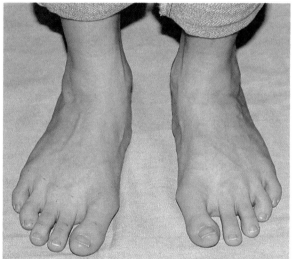

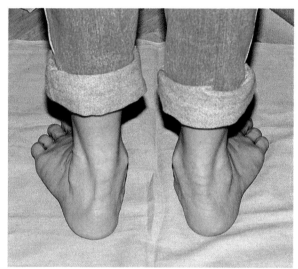

190–193 Identical twin girls of 11 years (**190** and **191**, and **192** and **193**, respectively) with **pronated feet and everted heels**. The forefeet are abducted. There is early hallux valgus, and rotation of the 4th and 5th toes. Footwear is good, and there is no clear family history of this condition.

7 Local manifestations of systemic disease

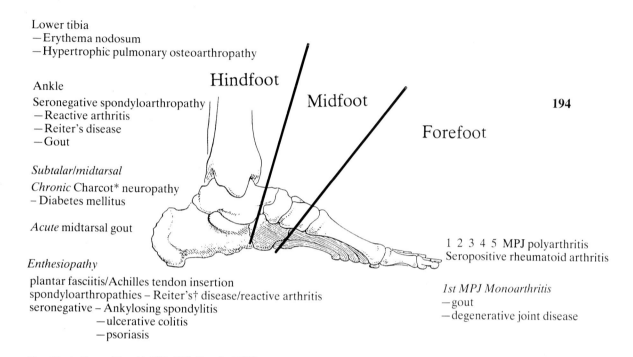

Lower tibia
—Erythema nodosum
—Hypertrophic pulmonary osteoarthropathy

Hindfoot

Midfoot

194

Ankle
Seronegative spondyloarthropathy
—Reactive arthritis
—Reiter's disease
—Gout

Forefoot

Subtalar/midtarsal
Chronic Charcot* neuropathy
– Diabetes mellitus

Acute midtarsal gout

1 2 3 4 5 MPJ polyarthritis
Seropositive rheumatoid arthritis

Enthesiopathy
plantar fasciitis/Achilles tendon insertion
spondyloarthropathies – Reiter's† disease/reactive arthritis
seronegative – Ankylosing spondylitis
　　　　　—ulcerative colitis
　　　　　—psoriasis

1st MPJ Monoarthritis
—gout
—degenerative joint disease

Jean Martin Charcot (French), 1825–1893. Described 1868
†*Hans Conrad Reiter* (German), 1881–1969. Described 1916

'. . . and Asa in the thirty ninth year of his reign was diseased in his feet, until his disease was exceeding great: yet in his disease he sought not to the Lord, but to the physicians . . .'.

(Asa, King of Judah, died in the 41st year of his reign) *Chronicles* 16, 12.

Site of pain

Locating the site of pain may suggest the likely group of disease involved, and so prompt examination of another part of the body.

Ask yourself:

Is it a monoarthritis or polyarthritis?
Is it a symmetrical polyarthritis?

What is the site? Are there other systemic manifestations?

Acute monoarthritis

- Infections: *Staphylococcus, Streptococcus,* Gram-negative organisms
- Crystal induced inflammation
  urate: foot-gout
  calcium pyrophosphate: knee-pseudogout
- Other inflammatory arthritides.
- Trauma

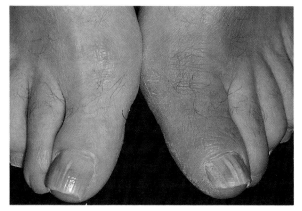

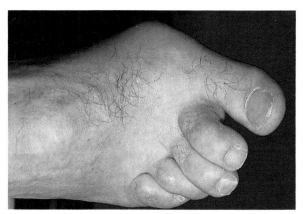

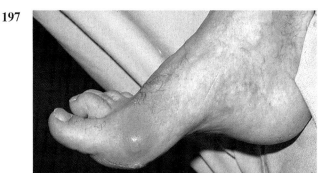

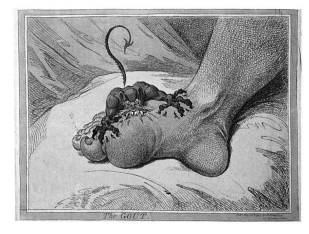

The GOUT.

followed by desquamation (**200**). Linear yellow discoloration in the nail of the great toe (**195**) suggests fungal infection.

The Gilray cartoon of 1799 (**198**) graphically portrays the symptomatology.

199 Midtarsal gout presents as a sudden severe pain in the midtarsus, accompanied by swelling, and a *pitting oedema* which continued for three weeks. A common variant of urate crystal synovitis, its dramatic onset often leads to it being confused with other conditions, infection sometimes being suspected. An American geologist awoke with pain in the midtarsus, the severity of which convinced him that he must have broken something. He referred himself to a radiologist for an X-ray. No firm diagnosis was made for three weeks.

The patient is usually a post-pubertal male, who may have had an elevated serum uric acid for four to five decades. The first attack usually affects the 1st MPJ, followed, in descending frequency, by the midtarsus, ankle, heel, knee, wrist and elbow.

195–198 Acute gout—podagra ('Greek foot trap', alluding to a man trap)—presents overnight as a sudden onset of severe pain in the great toe. So exquisitely tender is it that, on waking from sleep, the sufferer is unable even to bear a sheet upon it. The vivid inflammation is followed by swelling, which may last for seven to 14 days, to be

200 Desquamation of the skin of the forefoot at the defervescence of a 21-day attack of undiagnosed acute gout. Acute gout inflammation and bacterial inflammation may both desquamate as they remit.

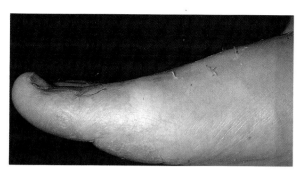

Chronic tophaceous gout

Sodium urate crystals may be deposited in the tissues—in the cartilage of the ear, around the elbow or foot, and in the kidney as calculi. Their appearance may be characteristic; a clue is the chalky appearance seen through the underlying skin, although the site may lead to confusion with other conditions. Tophi may discharge or become secondarily infected; they are usually painless.

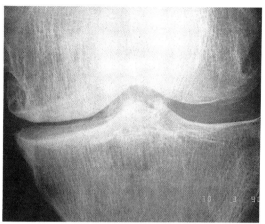

201

X-ray of the knee

Pseudogout (calcium pyrophosphate crystal synovitis) is clinically identical to gout. Usually, it affects the knee or wrist in males in their sixth or seventh decade. Associated with chondrocalcinosis, it is seen on X-ray as calcification in cartilage (**201**). Cartilage calcifications are seen also in diseases associated with divalent metals:

Ca++   —hyperparathyroidism
Cu++   —Wilson's disease
Fe++   —haemochromatosis
Mg++   —hypomagnesaemia

—as well as gout and degenerative joint disease.

201 X-ray of knee showing **calcification** in cartilage – **chondrocalcinosis**.

202–204 A tophus in the ear, presenting as a white/yellow substance under the skin which can be extruded (**204**).

203

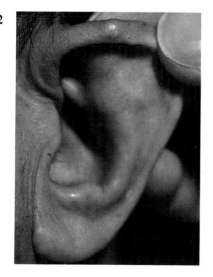

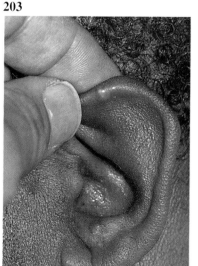

204

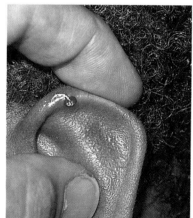

205

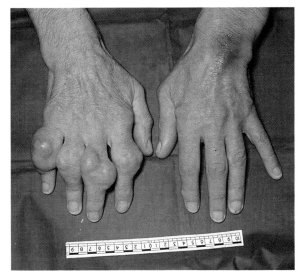

205 Tophi affecting the right hand. Swellings overlie the proximal interphalangeal (IP) joints; these must not be confused with the osteophytes of degenerative joint disease (Bouchard's nodes). Typical yellow translucent urate is seen over the right little finger, and this is the clue to the diagnosis. There is marked wasting of the first dorsal interosseus muscle and a bruise from venepuncture.

206

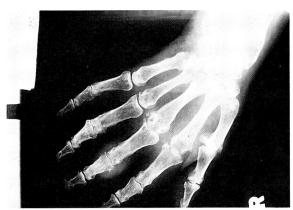

206 Gouty tophus. An X-ray showing **asymmetric soft tissue swelling** about the proximal IP joint of the middle finger. The swelling is radiolucent, gouty tophi rarely being calcified. Erosions are produced on the margins of bone away from the joint surface. Deposits appearing as radiolucent ovals can be seen in the proximal phalanx. Osteophytes are not present, nor is there osteoporosis.

207

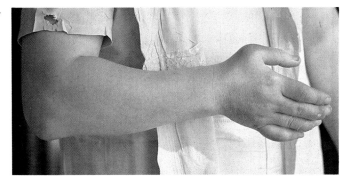

207 Chronic tophaceous gout. Tophi are present at the olecranon, mimicking a bursa, and over the base of the thumb, the terminal IP joint of the middle and ring fingers, and the proximal IP joint of the little finger. Urate is extruding through the skin and desquamation is seen over the middle finger.

208 Chronic tophaceous gout of the terminal phalanx—a recent acute attack that is still red and inflamed.

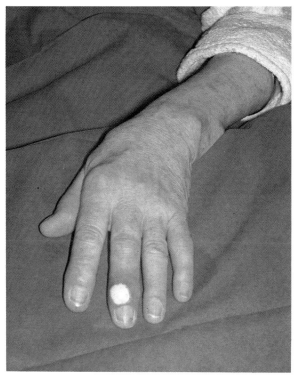

209 Chronic tophaceous gout of the feet. Tophi may occur around the great toe and be mistaken for osteophytes or bursae—the yellow urate can be seen through the skin. A tophus is present at the base of the 5th toe.

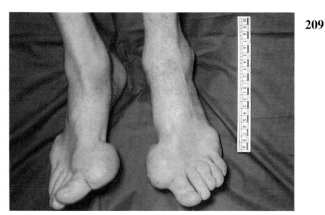

210 Infected discharging tophi of the feet. A tophus overlies the lateral part of the great toe and urate is discharging from a tophus over the middle toe. Treatment continued for many weeks before the underlying gout was appreciated.

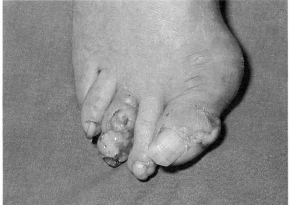

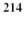

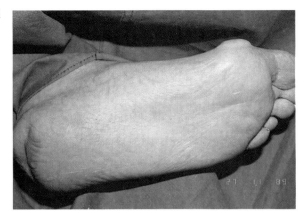

211 and 212 A gouty tophus over the lateral side of the great toe. Note the healed scar of a bed sore on the heel, acquired ten years earlier. Such scars with fibrotic tethering and loss of fibro-fatty padding are often a long-term problem at this site.

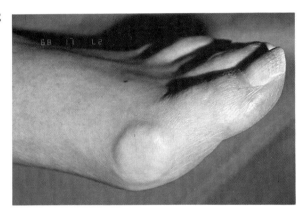

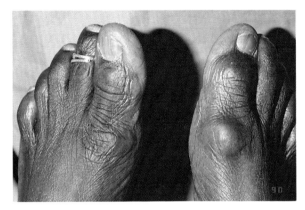

213 Osteoarthritis and hallux rigidus. By contrast, the osteophyte produced this prominence over the dorso-lateral area of the right first MPJ. Note the toe ring which was worn inside the subject's normal footwear.

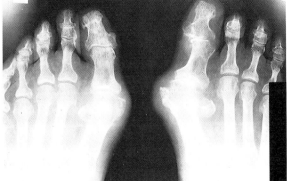

214 Tophaceous gout, in an X-ray of the feet. There is usually little osteophyte formation in gout; and any bony erosion in the feet may be masked if co-existing with degenerative joint disease, since the latter leads to osteophytes around the IP joint of the great toe. Erosions are present at the lateral side of the right great toe.

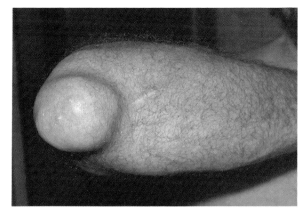

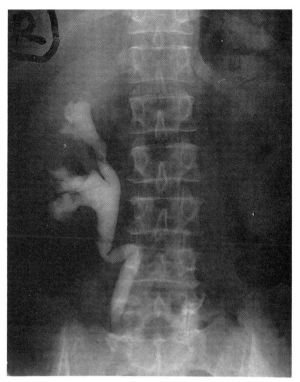

215 A gouty tophus at the olecranon. Despite urate being visible through the skin, this was thought to be a simple olecranon bursitis.

216 Intravenous urogram urate calculi. Urate calculi may produce obstruction and a hydronephrosis of the ureter and kidney, though the actual calculus is radiolucent. Large urate stones may be present in the renal pelvis and yet be overlooked unless care is exercised.

Polyarthritis

Symmetrical small joint involvement of the feet and hands may be seen in rheumatoid arthritis and other connective tissue diseases. Differentiation will depend on the clinical picture, the presence of rheumatoid factor, and the involvement of the other systems. Though deformities of the hands resulting from seropositive rheumatoid arthritis may be typical, those of the feet may be less so, due to joint-ligament erosion and joint destruction. In the feet the main pain problem is pain on weight-bearing. Early rheumatoid arthritis and other seronegative polyarthropathies may produce a similar appearance.

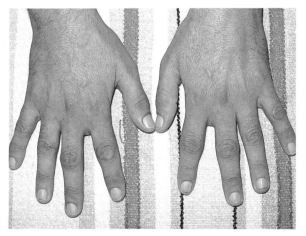

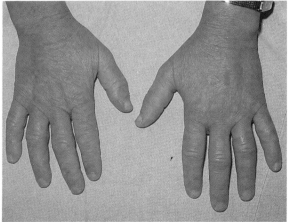

217 Early acute rheumatoid arthritis. There is swelling of the proximal IP joints, which is particularly marked in the index, middle and ring fingers.

218 Polyarthritis—systemic lupus and erythematosus swelling of all the IP joints, with less obvious spindling.

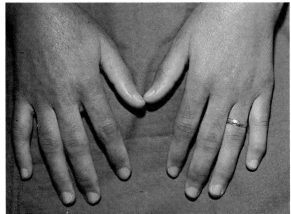

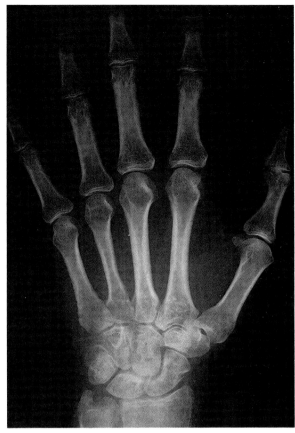

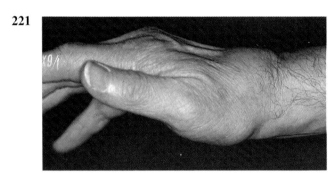

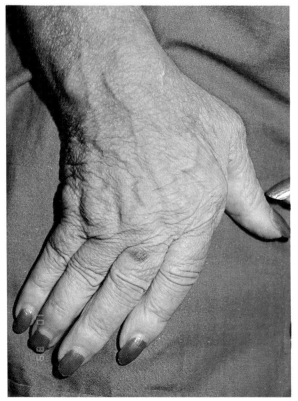

219 A seronegative polyarthritis with swelling of the IP joints and shiny stiff skin, in a woman with mixed connective tissue disease.

220 An X-ray of a hand with **early seropositive rheumatoid arthritis.** Periarticular osteoporosis and soft tissue swelling are both present. Very early joint erosions. An initial increase in joint space may occur due to synovial effusion, later decreasing as cartilage is lost.

221 Rheumatoid arthritis. Swelling of the wrist is due to synovial thickening and effusion in the carpus, with limitation of movement. There is wasting of the interossei with guttering, secondary to the inflammatory arthritis.

222 Rheumatoid arthritis—ulnar deviation. The ulnar drift of the finger is due to erosion of the ligaments. The purpuric spot at the base of the middle finger reflects capillary fragility and steroid therapy.

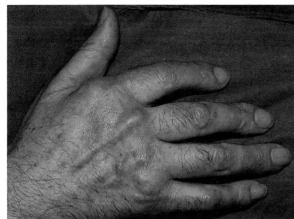

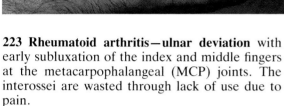

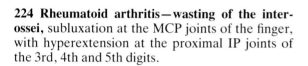

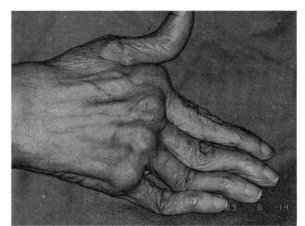
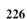

223 Rheumatoid arthritis—ulnar deviation with early subluxation of the index and middle fingers at the metacarpophalangeal (MCP) joints. The interossei are wasted through lack of use due to pain.

224 Rheumatoid arthritis—wasting of the interossei, subluxation at the MCP joints of the finger, with hyperextension at the proximal IP joints of the 3rd, 4th and 5th digits.

225–227 A trio of hands with a spectrum of deformity: moderately advanced **rheumatoid arthritis with ulnar deviation.** Swelling at the IP joints, particularly at the proximal IP joints, is a characteristic sign (**226**). MCP subluxation with a Z-deformity of the thumbs, swan neck deformity of the index finger and boutonnière deformity of the middle finger of the left hand are also seen (**227**).

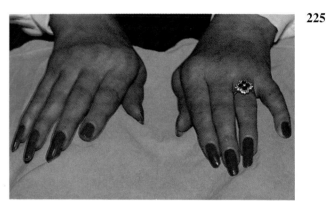

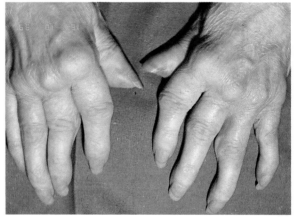

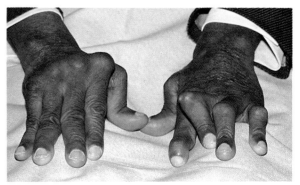

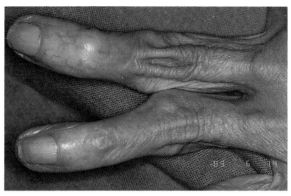

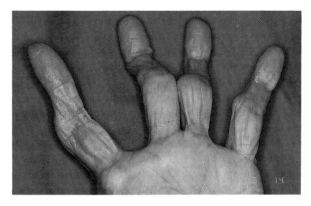

230

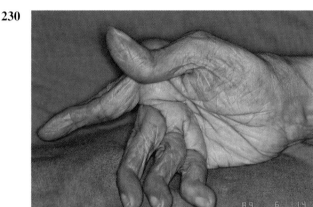

231

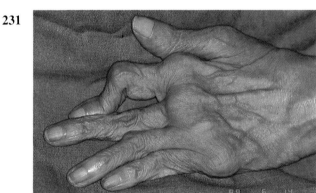

232

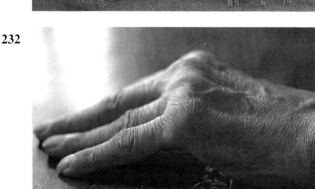

228 Swan neck deformity—rheumatoid arthritis. Hyperextension at the proximal IP joint with flexion at the terminal IP joint. Forward sub-luxation of the MCP joint causes the intrinsic muscles to be tightened, which in turn causes the MCP to flex as finger extension occurs—but if there is destruction of the volar plate of the proximal IP joint, the hyperextension occurs here. The distal IP joint is flexed because the pull of the extended profundus tendon exceeds that of the long extensor tendon, two lateral slips of which can be seen bowstrung across the proximal IP joints.

229 Boutonnière (buttonhole) deformity of the index finger, contrasting with swan neck deformity of the lateral three digits.

230 Z-shaped deformity of the thumb—hitch-hiker's thumb. Damage to the MCP joint causes the long and short extensors to be displaced volar wards on the ulnar side of the thumb, leading to loss of extension at the MCP joint and hyper-extension at the IP joint occurs from tension of the long thumb extensor. The remainder of the digits exhibit varying degrees of swan neck deformity. There is wasting of the thenar eminence.

Buttonhole/boutonnière mechanism: if the inflammation at the proximal IP joint causes damage to, and destruction of, the central slip of the extensor insertion into the base of the middle phalanx, the proximal IP joint may then protrude between the lateral extensions of the extensor tendon, producing the 'button through a button hole'—or boutonnière—deformity with the extensions acting as flexors across this joint.

231 Buttonhole deformity of the index fingers. With subluxation of the MCP joints and swan neck deformity of the lateral three digits, the interossei are wasted (**232**).

233 An X-ray of the hand in a case of **late rheumatoid arthritis.** The loss of joint space is due to the destruction of cartilage and to juxta-articular osteoporosis and erosions.

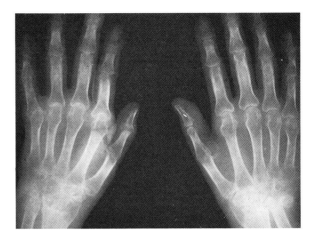

Soft tissue changes in the plantar surface of the forefoot in rheumatoid arthritis

234–237 Discrete swellings over the metatarsal (MT) heads (**234–236**) and the proximal part of half of the great toe (**237**) are produced by a bursitis or cyst formation leading to the complaint of 'walking on pebbles'. Occasionally, small sinuses occur at the apex of these swellings (**234, 237, 239**). Where the swellings occur there is separation of the dermal ridges (**236**). There is usually little or no callus formation over the swellings.

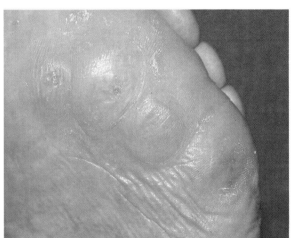

234

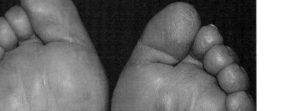

235

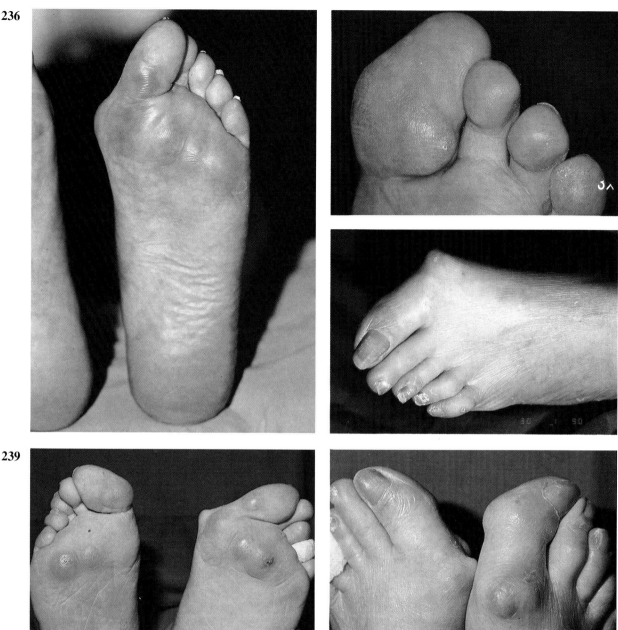

238–240 Later changes may include **fibular drift** (compare with ulnar drift in **222**) **of all the toes** at the MTP joints (**238**). The great toe may even lie near to a right angle to the 1st mt. Shiny pale thin skin may reflect the steroid therapy, and there is an absence of dorsal skin creases in association with the joints (**238**). A sinus overlies the bursa associated with the left and right 4th mt heads (**239**). There is a rheumatoid nodule at the base of the right first toe (**240**).

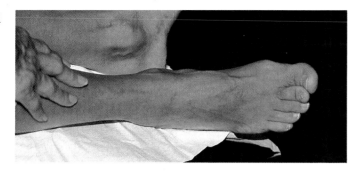

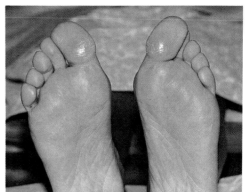

241 and 242 The **rheumatoid deformity** in the hand contrasts with the absence of stigmata on the dorsal foot, belying the appearance of the plantar surface where there are typical soft tissue changes (**242**) on the proximal great toe.

243 and 244 Rheumatoid arthritis. The right foot (**243**) shows mild soft tissue changes over the 2nd and 4th mt heads, with fibular drift of the 2nd and 3rd toes in parallel with the ageing change in a shod foot. The left great toe has a marked hallux valgus deformity and some rotation with fibular drift of the 2nd and 3rd toes (**244**). There is soft tissue swelling under the 2nd and 4th mt heads and less so under the 1st (**244**).

243

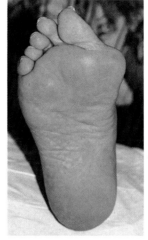

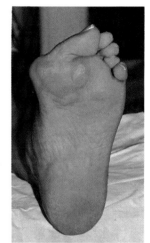

244

245 Rheumatoid arthritis—the only soft tissue change is a bursa seen in profile on the medial/dorsal border. The 2nd toe is displaced dorsally.

245

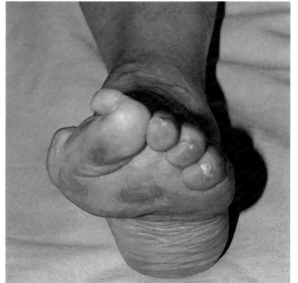

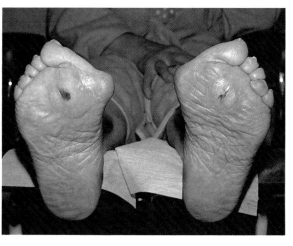

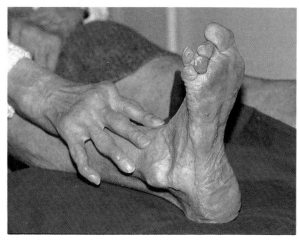

246 Rheumatoid hallux valgus with soft tissue changes over the 2nd and 3rd mt heads, which have uncharacteristic callus formation and pale thin shiny skin over the great toes.

247 Atrophy of the whole of the soft tissues on the plantar surface, in long-term steroid therapy for rheumatoid arthritis.

Systemic manifestations of rheumatoid arthritis

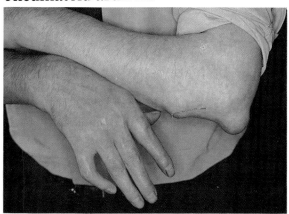

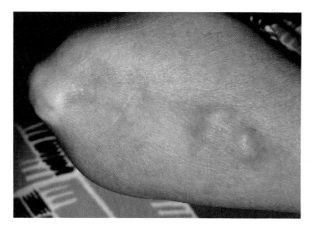

248–250 Rheumatoid nodules consist of granulomatous tissue and may necrose. Found subcutaneously in association with bony or tendinous prominences (**249 and 250**), they are frequently seen in seropositive individuals. They may be found around the occiput and the Achilles tendon, or be present in many other tissues. The differential diagnosis may include gouty tophi, bursae, synovial cysts, xanthomata, neurofibromata etc.

248 Rheumatoid hand shows ulnar deviation of the fingers at the metacarpophalangeal joints, early dislocation of the little finger at the MCP joint, but no evidence of IP joint swelling— a heavy smoker (witness the nicotine-stained fingers). There is synovial thickening in the right wrist. A left olecranon bursa and a rheumatoid nodule along the subcutaneous border of the ulnar are also present.

251 Rheumatoid nodule overlying the ischial tuberosity and another of the sacrum where necrosis, infection and breakdown have occurred.

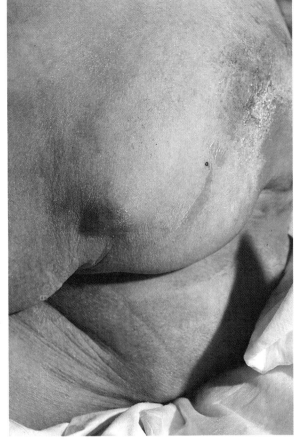

251

252–257 Vasculitis. The appearance of nail fold vasculitis (**252** to **254**) may be associated with splinter haemorrhages in the nail. This appearance may be an indication of the presence of IgM immunoglobulins and seropositivity. Ischaemic vasculitis may lead to necrosis and ulceration (**255–257**).

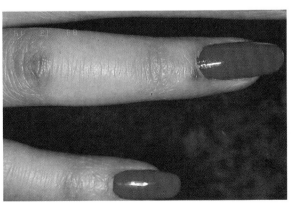

252

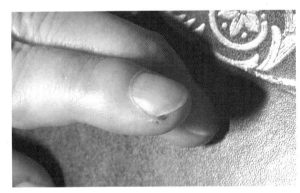

253

254

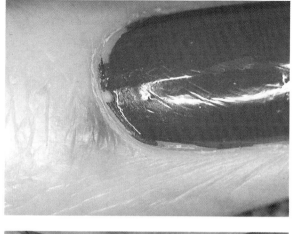

2

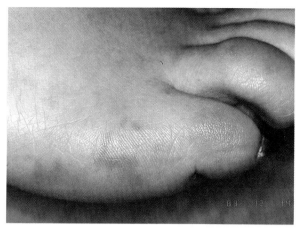

256

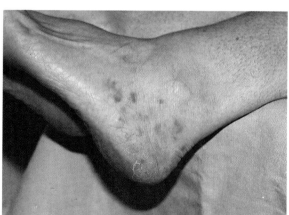

2

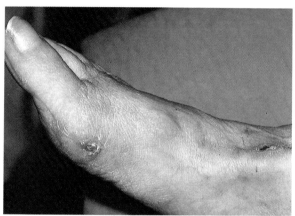

258

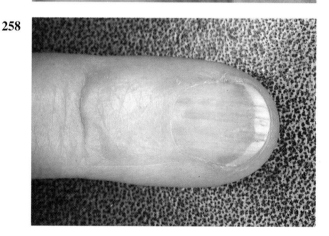

258 Ridging and beading of the nail is often seen in the elderly. Their association with rheumatoid arthritis may be of little significance.

Seronegative polyarthritis

In the differential diagnosis of polyarthritis a broad distinction can be drawn between seropositive polyarthritis with the presence of rheumatoid factor and a large group of other connective tissue diseases which have poly or oligo arthritis as a feature but are usually seronegative. Manifestations in the feet produce pain and deformity; some of the clinical presentations are distinctive.

Progressive systemic sclerosis: facies

259 An English woman aged 60 years, with tight facial skin and a typical puckered mouth with radiating skin creases. There is **telangiectasia** over the face; this can be difficult to see in non-Caucasian skins. The skin of the hands is taut and telangiectatic, but no terminal phalanx absorption or nail changes are visible.

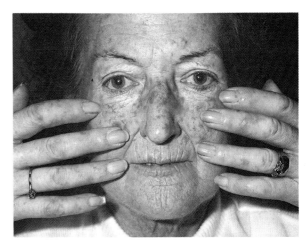

260 A Sudanese woman of 60 years, with tight facial skin with perioral, orbital and thoracic thickening and depigmentation. The lower lip has been tattooed and decorative scars are seen on the cheeks.

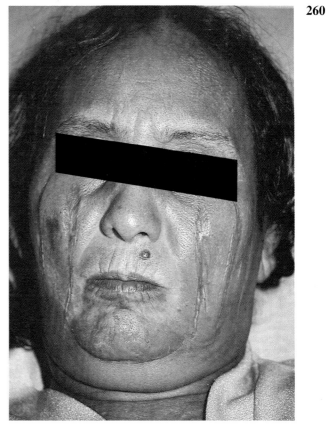

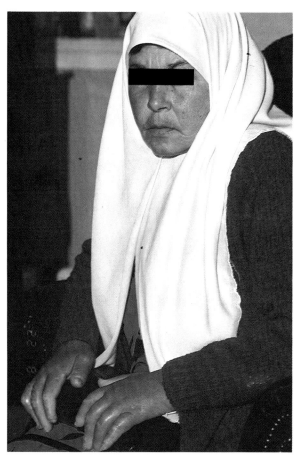

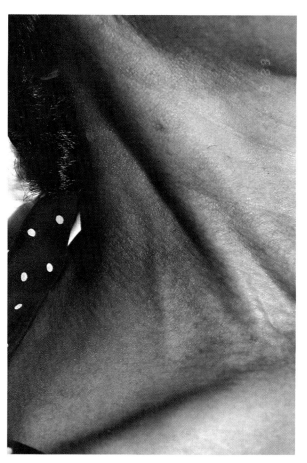

261 and 262 A Palestinian woman aged 50 years with minimal facial changes, although the labial changes are apparent. The skin of the hands is tight and shiny, and severely affected (**268**). Her neck (**262**) shows patchy depigmentation.

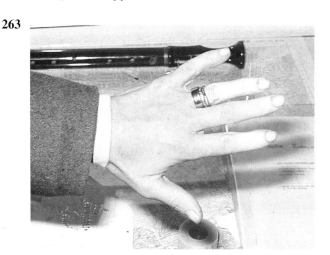

263 Raynaud's phenomenon in an English domestic cleaner. She has arrived on a cold morning with white vasoconstricted fingers and has not yet removed her top coat. In a few minutes the fingers flush with returning blood flow. Three years later she developed progressive systemic sclerosis.

Severe Raynaud's phenomenon may precede later changes by several years, however. The cleaning lady developed facial changes, peripheral arthritis, dyspnoea from lung involvement and dysphagia from oesophageal hypomotility. Her oesophagus is seen in **278**.

264 Early seronegative polyarthritis in systemic sclerosis. The skin is taut and shiny but no other changes are seen.

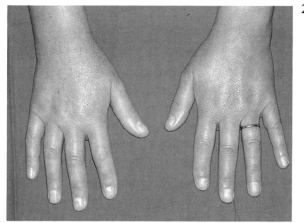

Late progressive systemic sclerosis (PSS) affecting the extremities

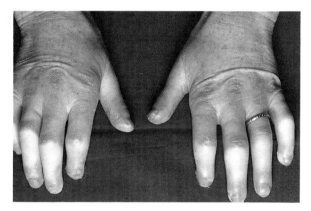

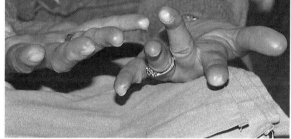

265 and 266 Hands with tight blanched skin of the fingers and dorsum (**265**) with terminal phalangeal resorption and pseudo clubbing (**266**).

267 Nail pulp infarcts in systemic sclerosis. The scars of these vasculitic infarcts are prominent on the index and ring fingers.

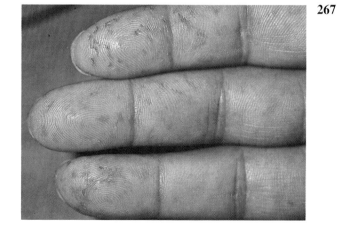

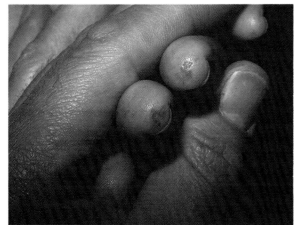

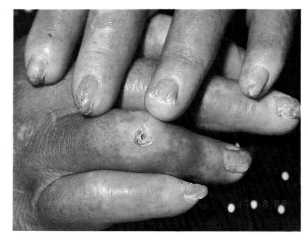

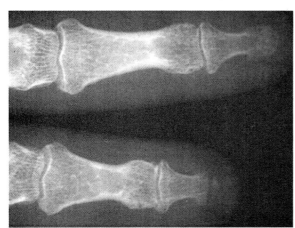

268 Terminal phalangeal resorption occurs and may be associated with extrusion of a calcified material. The sinuses where this has occurred have closed on two fingertips.

269 Systemic sclerosis, tight skin, atrophy of subcutaneous tissue, depigmentation, nail dystrophy, terminal phalangeal resorption with curling of the nail around the tip of the left index and middle fingers (pseudo clubbing). Ulceration over the middle phalanx of the ring finger may be mirrored in the feet (**275**). The little finger is tapered due to the effect of osteolysis of its terminal phalanx. A picture of sclerodactyly.

270 An X-ray showing loss of terminal phalangeal bone. The acronym CREST describes the clinical picture:
C = calcinosis subcutaneous calcium often
   extruded;
R = Raynaud's phenomenon;
E = esophageal hypomotility;
S = sclerodactyly; and
T = telangiectasia.

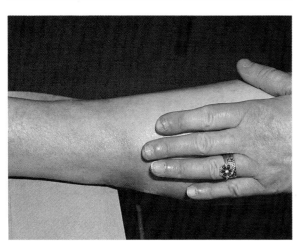

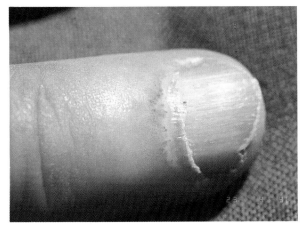

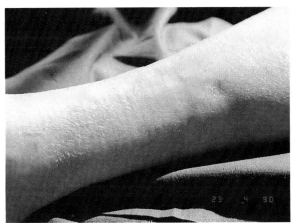

271–274 The skin of the leg (**271**) shows a clear demarcation below which the subcutaneous tissue is absent and the skin thickened, tethered and shiny. Telangiectasia often affects the face, and nail fold capillary loops become prominent (**272**), with hyperkeratotic irregular cuticles overlapping with the appearance in dermatomyositis. Ridging and beading of the nail is present. The change in subcutaneous tissue extends to the plantar surface (**274**), with telangiectatic thin skin and the loss of fibro-fatty padding.

275 On the dorsum the skin is leathery, tethered and pigmented, the nails dystrophic. The toes contrast with the hands (**269**).

276 Peripheral cyanosis and cold intolerance with chilblains are a problem.

274

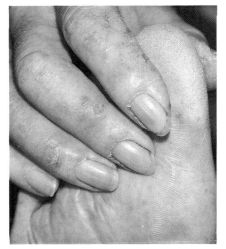

276

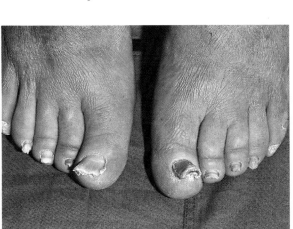

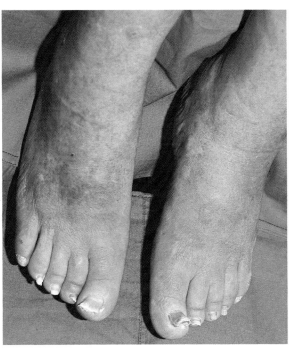

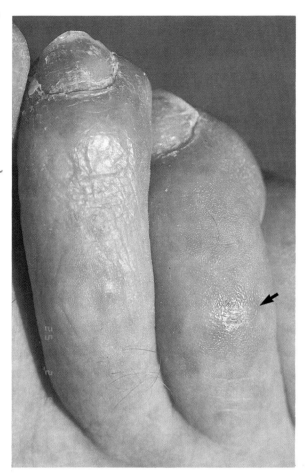

277 Localised ulceration of the digits may occur on the toes as in the hands (**269**).

Other systemic manifestations of PSS

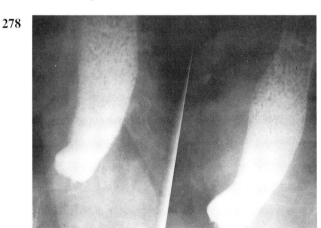

278 Barium meal: oesophageal hypomotility. After the skin and the joints, the gut comes next in frequency of involvement in this multisystem disease. It occurs late in the course—involvement of the distal two thirds of the oesophagus produces hypomobility and poor emptying, with dilation and widening with reflux of barium in the oesophagus, which has lost its normal mobility. Fibrosis of the lung may lead to disturbances of gaseous interchange and renal and cardiac involvement to system failure.

PSS may affect the joints, gut, lungs, heart and kidney, as well as the skin—compared with localised scleroderma or morphea, which has a quite different prognosis.

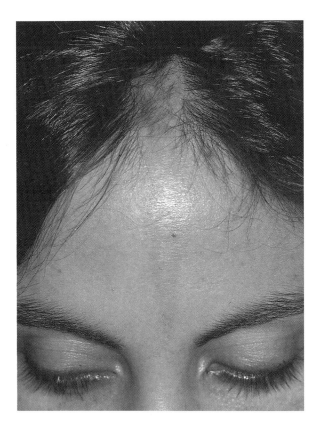

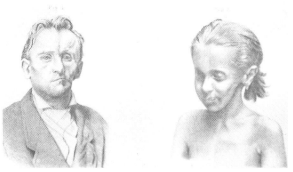

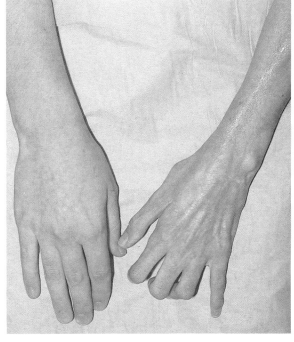

281

279–281 Localised scleroderma or *coup de sabre* (so called because of its alleged similarity to a sabre-cut scar). There is linear pigmentation and subcutaneous atrophy extending into the hair line with local alopecia. It may be gross (**280**)* and associated with hemifacial and limb atrophy (**281**).

282 and 283 Subcutaneous localised scleroderma and atrophy and tethering became worse in childhood but remained stationary after the age of 12. Thin shiny atrophic skin (**282**) with areas of thickening and pigmentation (**283**) are also seen.

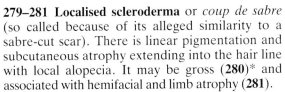
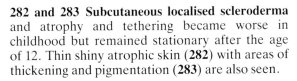

‵2

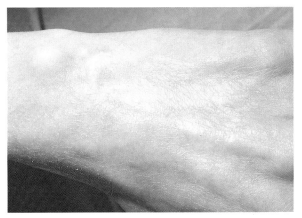

283

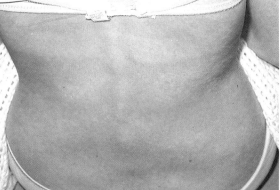

Archives of Surgery, Jonathan Hutchinson

Pain in the heel

This may be due to a local mechanical cause or to overuse, or it may be a manifestation of a sero-negative spondyloarthropathy.

Causes

- Overuse—bursitis.
- Weight—plantar fasciitis.
- Osteochondritis calcaneum—seven- to 13-year-old male.
- Trauma of heel.
- Infection.
- Juvenile arthritis and ankle pain.
- Osteoid osteoma.
- Seronegative spondyloarthropathies.

Seronegative spondyloarthropathies comprise a group of disorders having in common degrees of sacroilitis, spondylitis and peripheral arthritis, and sharing increased-frequency of genetic markers as well as X-ray changes. Included are ankylosing spondylitis, reactive arthritis (Reiter's syndrome), psoriatic arthritis, and the spondylitis associated with gastrointestinal conditions such as Crohn's* disease and ulcerative colitis. All may show enthesiopathies—inflammation at the site of insertion of tendons into bone or fascia—which may produce heel pain as well as inflammatory disease of the spine and sacroiliac joints, and peripheral, often oligo, arthritis, usually affecting large joints. Extra-articular involvement with uveitis, aortitis and the skin may occur. The HLA 27 antigen is strongly associated.

Immunological reactions to infection which produce a reactive arthritis may be associated with the HLA B27 histocompatibility antigen; the infections may be enteric or venereal, and include shigella, salmonella, yersinia or campylobacter infections. In non-HLA B27 associated disease, post-streptococcal manifestations such as rheumatic fever and Henoch–Schönlein purpura may occur. In reactive arthritis the clinical picture encompasses an asymmetric or oligo arthritis as well as the urethritis, conjunctivitis, circinate balanitis, plantar fasciitis and keratoderma blenorrhagica which may be similar in appearance to pustular psoriasis.

In ankylosing spondylitis and reactive arthritis heel pain may occur. While this is usually felt on the plantar surface, it may be localised to the enthesium.

*Burrill Bernard Crohn (US), 1884–19??

284

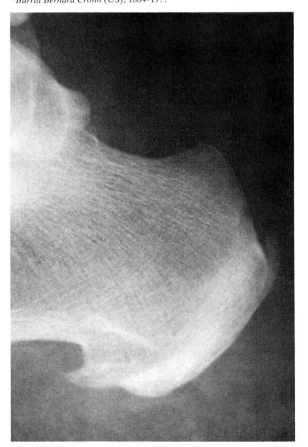

284 Plantar spur: X-ray of heel. At the insertion of the Achilles tendon and the plantar fascia into the calcaneum (the enthesium) can be seen spurs of calcium where ossification of the enthesium has occurred. Changes may include soft tissue swelling and erosions, as well as spur formation. In reactive arthritis periostitis may be a striking feature. Plantar spurs in Reiter's disease may be large and fluffy and associated with heel pain, although they may be asymptomatic.

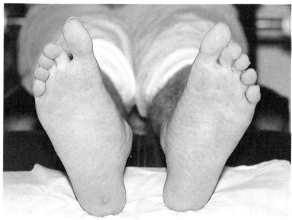

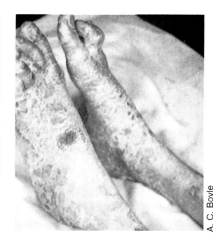

A. C. Boyle

285 Sub-talar joint involvement in reactive arthritis (Reiter's). Both feet have tipped into valgus, more so on the right. There is a scar extending to the 3rd cleft on the left foot where a digital neuroma has been excised.

286 and 287 Keratoderma blenorrhagica (286) — compare with pustular psoriasis (**287**). It may appear within one month of the precipitating infection and consists of a papulo-vesicular rash which may desquamate or form plaques. Palms or soles may be affected.

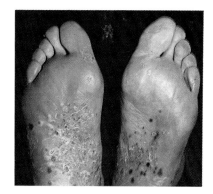

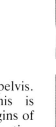

288 and 289 Ankylosing spondylitis. This seronegative spondyloarthropathy has sacro-iliac and spinal joint involvement. The X-ray (**289**) shows calcification of the anterior spinal ligament producing the 'bamboo spine'. There is severe limitation of movement at the neck and a horizontal visual axis is possible only by hyperextension at the atlanto-occipital articulation with the skull (**289**).

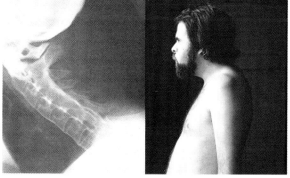

290 Ankylosing spondylitis: X-ray of pelvis. Sacro-iliac ankylosis has occurred. This is preceded by resorption of the cortical margins of the sacrum and ilium. Multiple areas of reactive trabecular bone surround the widened irregular joint space.

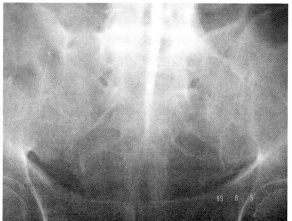

286

287

288
289

290

Psoriatic arthropathy

Psoriatic arthropathy affects seven per cent of psoriatic patients, usually in the fourth or fifth decade (compared to the skin manifestations which appear in the second or third). It is an asymmetrical oligo arthritis affecting the distal IP joints of the hands and feet.

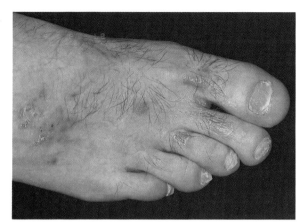

291 Psoriatic plaques on the dorsum of the foot and 1st, 2nd and 3rd toes. They are red, irregular, and sharply defined, with overlying silver scales which, if scraped away, may show red bleeding points of hypertrophied dermal papillae. There is nail dystrophy of all toes, but no joint involvement. The plaques are seen on extensor surfaces, pressure areas, natal cleft, navel, penis and scalp. They may appear in scars and on areas of trauma (Koebner's* phenomenon: linear trauma).

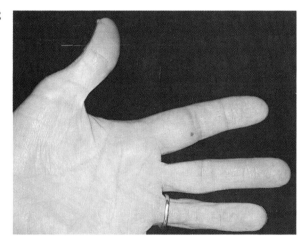

292 There may be a sausage-shaped swelling of the finger due to distal and proximal IP (as well as MCP) joint involvement of the same finger or toe, associated with a flexor tenosynovitis.

A similar appearance can occur in the short term due to gout, trauma, or sickle cell disease bone infarct, and in the long term due to gouty tophi, sarcoid bone cysts (look for lupus pernio), Ollier's disease (enchondroplasia), and chronic inflammation such as tuberculosis and syphilitic gummata, as well as psoriasis.

In 15% of psoriatic arthropathies there may be a seronegative symmetrical polyarthritis indistinguishable from rheumatoid arthritis, and usually seen in women.

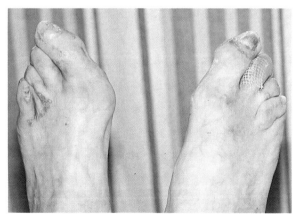

293 Psoriasis and psoriatic arthropathy of the feet. On the right middle and left middle and 5th toes there are psoriatic skin lesions with characteristic red plaques with overlying silver scale. There is thickening and yellow discoloration of the right great toe nail, and hallux valgus with IP joint swelling and midtarsal swelling of the right foot.

Heinreich Koebner (German), 1838–1944

294 An X-ray of the left foot. There is a pencil-in-cup deformity of the 4th IP joint with characteristic proliferative erosion of the proximal phalanx.

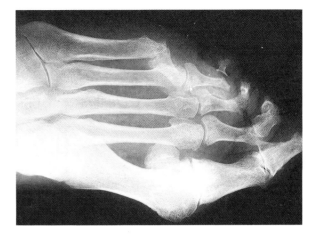

295 An X-ray of the right foot. Loss of joint space in the IP joint is best seen in the great toe.

A predominantly distal IP-joint arthritis associated with nail involvement may occur in ten per cent of these individuals; it may be asymmetric.

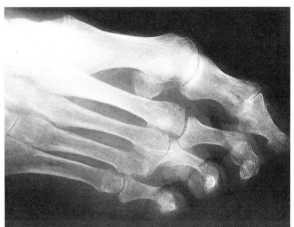

296 There is pitting and onycholysis on the right index finger, and there are nail pits in the ring and left little finger nails. There is also swelling of the IP and MCP joints, with interosseus wasting—seen as guttering on the back of the hand.

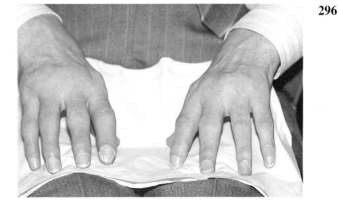

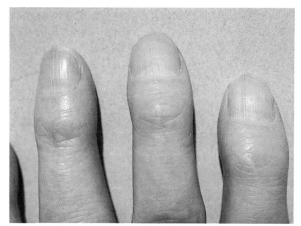

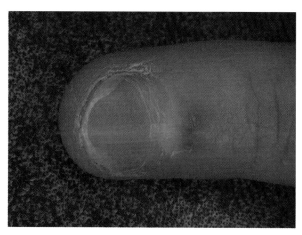

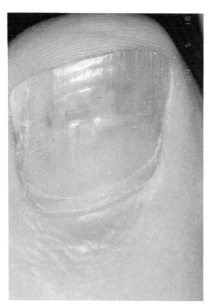

299

297 Terminal IP swelling and pitting of the nail on the index finger. There is ridging and beading of the nail. An axial spondyloarthropathy with low backache may occur in five per cent of cases.

298 Onycholyis of the finger nail.

299 Onycholysis of the great toe nail. In addition to psoriasis, causes of onycholysis include fungal and candida infection, trauma, ischaemia, thyroid disease, dermatitis, and the yellow nail syndrome. There is also an idiopathic variety.

A deforming erosive arthritis may occur in less than five per cent of cases. Though uncommon, this is always remembered by the student as a result of its distinctive, if unattractive, name: arthritis mutilans. Terminal IP joint erosion and osteolysis occurs, and may lead to telescoping of fingers and toes.

300–303 Psoriasis—the lorgnette finger. This 70-year-old nun developed seronegative polyarthritis and, subsequently, nail changes of psoriasis of the hands and psoriasis of the scalp. The left little, middle and index fingers, as well as the right thumb, middle and ring fingers, show this sign (**300**). Onycholysis is present in the nail (**301**), and psoriatic arthritis is evident in **302** and **303**. Hallux valgus and osteolysis with telescoping of the 4th toe are also shown.

300

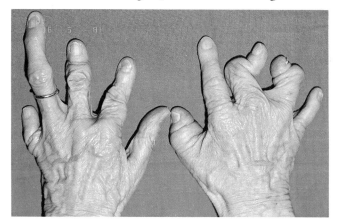

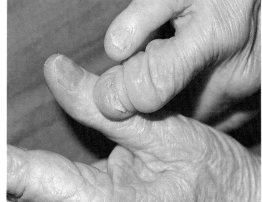

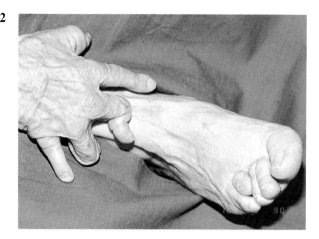
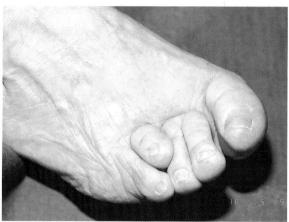

Soft tissue rheumatism

The origin of pain in the soft tissues about the feet may be:

- Capsule/ligament insertion.
- Tendon.
- Tendon sheath.
- Bursa.
- Fascia.

Pain may be associated with swelling, when the differential diagnosis may include neuromata, ganglia, xanthomata, and rheumatoid nodules. Pain may be precipitated by overuse and, in the obese, by prolonged standing.

Swelling may be due to occupational bursae resulting from repetitive trauma manifesting in complaints such as housemaid's knee and, in the coal miner, beat knee.

304 Achilles tendon bursitis. A rower developed pain in the tendon following very intensive practice. There is swelling around the left Achilles tendon due to inflammation of the superficial bursa following overuse. Typical transverse bruising at the junction of the middle and lower third of the calf is caused by the sliding seat of the boat at maximum limb flexion.

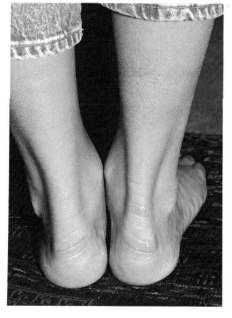

304

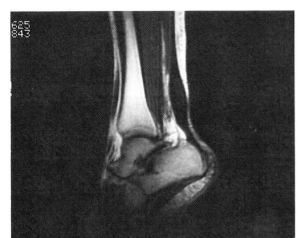

305 A nuclear magnetic resonance scan of an ankle shows the fusiform enlargement of the tendon in an overuse strain.

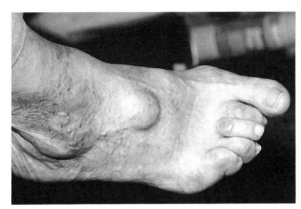

306 A ganglion on the dorsum of a (shoe-moulded) foot, seen in a male subject. Ganglia are cystic swellings of hyaluronate found near tendons, and are common on the dorsum. They may occur around the ankle behind the malleoli and compress the nerve. They transilluminate. On the dorsum, they are easily distinguished from exostoses which are bony.

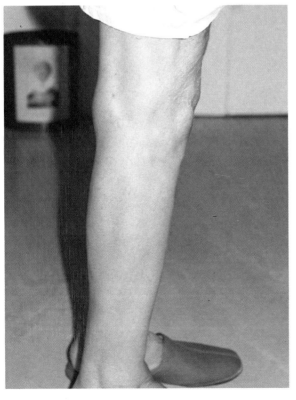

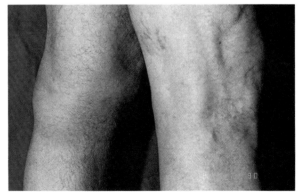

307–309 Baker's cyst. A cystic swelling behind the knee in the lower part of the popliteal fossa which is thrown into prominence on extension of the knee. It may rupture and cause pain and swelling. This syndrome of pseudothrombophlebitis presents with pain in the knee and an effusion—as well as pain, tenderness, swelling and redness in the calf; it may mimic a deep venous thrombosis or inflammatory arthritis, with which it may be associated. It occurs in LE, psoriasis, and ankylosing spondylitis, as well as in degenerative joint disease.

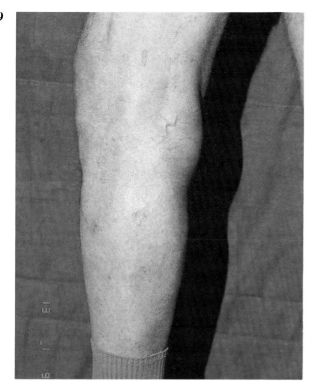

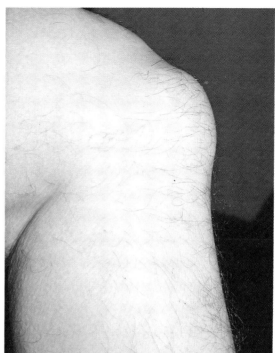

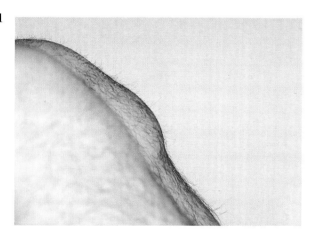

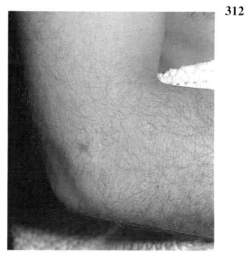

310 and 311 Infrapatellar bursitis. Bursae may be superficial or deep and become inflamed by trauma—particularly where this is repetitive and occupational. They may enlarge in rheumatic disease. The bursa here, seen in a clergyman, is similar to housemaid's knee.

312 Tennis elbow. Repetitive strain may produce pain at the insertion of the tendon, and the condition is not limited to tennis players! Here, the tattoo produced by an unpractised hand is minimised by the dermal atrophy of a local corticosteroid injection.

Other miscellaneous conditions

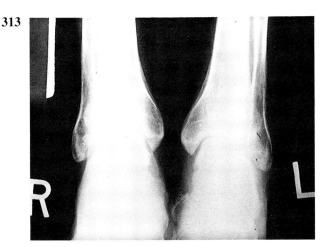

313

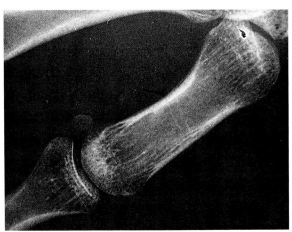

314

313 and 314 Hypertrophic pulmonary osteo-arthropathy, shown in an X-ray of the tibia. There is new bone formation due to periosteal reaction at the lower end of the tibia. This may also be seen in the bones of the forearm, and even in the long bone of the hand (**314**)—an arrow indicates the thin line of new bone formation running parallel to the long axis. This condition may be associated with pain in the limb and oedema. Nail clubbing is present. It may be the presenting feature of a carcinoma of the bronchus or it may complicate the course of cystic fibrosis.

Conditions which may deform the limb

315

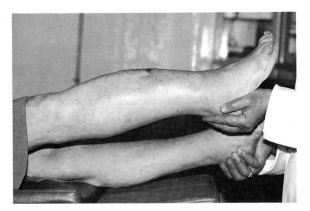

A change in the shape of the bone:

- Paget's disease.
- Rickets.

A local swelling:

- Enchondromata, exostoses, osteophytes, etc.

315 Paget's disease—osteitis deformans—in an elderly woman with increasing deafness and an aching lower leg. The tibia is bowed and expanded, as well as being warmer than the left. The disease is characterised by enlargement and deformity of bone.

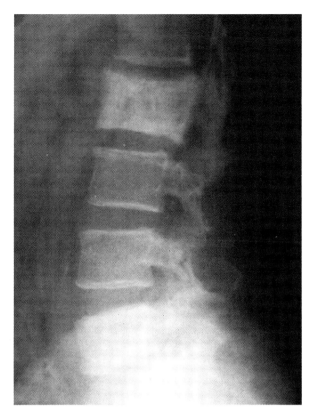

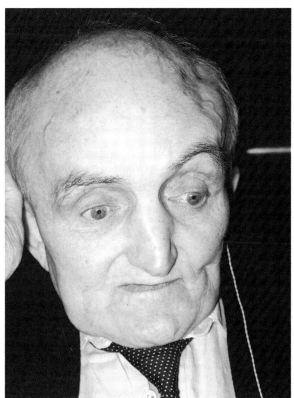

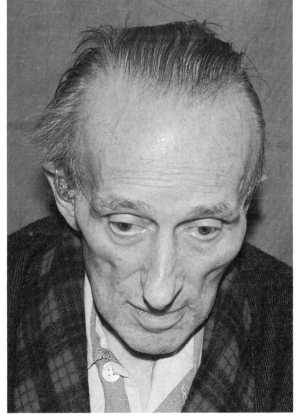

316 Paget's disease. An X-ray of the lumbar spine shows, radiologically, that there is an expansion and an increase in bone density—yet the bone may be hard and brittle.

317 and 318 Paget's disease. The skull is enlarged. If the expanded bone encroaches on an osseous foramen, it may compress the nerve that it encloses. Both subjects here have the condition, and become deaf (note the wire from the hearing aid in **317**) because of encroachment on the internal auditory meatus. A single bone may be affected or the condition may be polyostotic and affect the axial skeleton and weight-bearing bones.

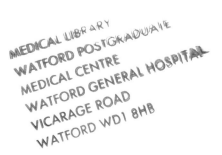

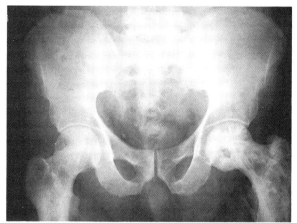

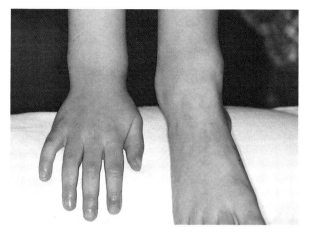

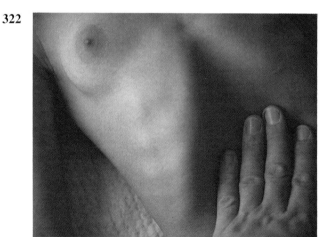

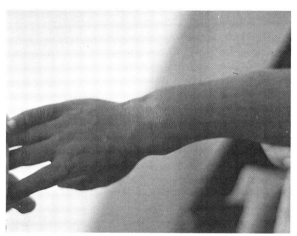

319 The left femur is affected by **Paget's disease**. This pagetic bone may ache or fracture. Complications locally include fracture, tumour, sarcoma, benign giant cell tumour, and reparative granuloma. Extramedullary haematopoiesis, and cardiac failure secondary to the shunt-induced high output state may occur.

320 Rickets. Before growth has ceased, deficiency of vitamin D leads to uncalcified osteoid tissue producing a widening of the zone between the epiphysis and metaphysis. The ankle and wrist are widened immediately above the joint and a second bump is seen above the malleoli and wrist crease. Wrist crease, too, is evident. The deficiency may be nutritional due to poor intake, or synthesis in the skin, malabsorption, renal disease due to inherited resistance to Vitamin D, and anti-convulsant therapy.

321 Rickets at the wrist.

322 Ricketty rosary, due to swelling at the costo-chondral junctions following increased deposition of osteoid tissue.

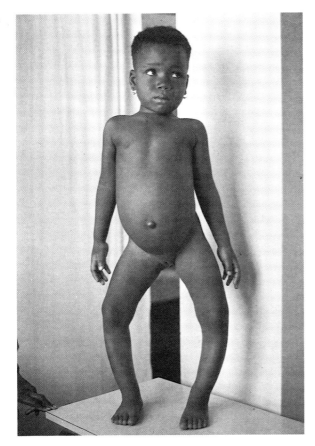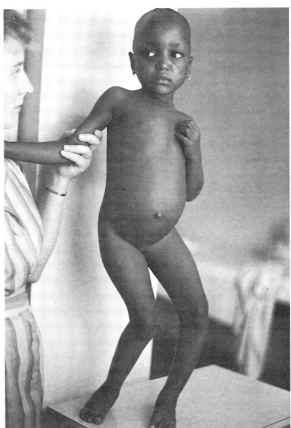

323 and 324 In the older child the mechanical stresses cause the soft tissue to bend and may lead to varus or valgus deformities.

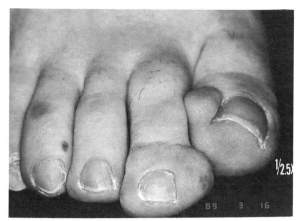

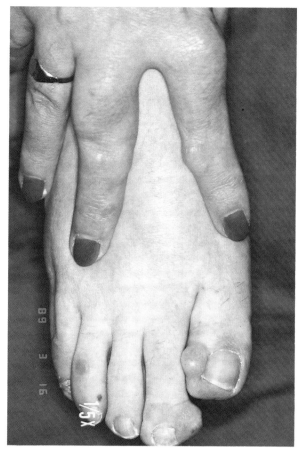

325 and 326 Enchondromatosis—Ollier's* disease.
Cartridge islands persist adjacent to the epiphyseal plate and produce disturbed growth with haemangiomata (2nd toe) which are often superficial (Maffucci† syndrome). This may be internal. The affected hands and feet are deformed by swellings adjacent to the joints and can be mistaken for arthritis. Cartridge islands expand the bone.

*Louis Xavier Ollier (French), 1830–1900
†Angelo Maffucci (Italian), 1845–1903. Described 1881

8 The swollen foot

The aim is to lead the student from the foot with its physical sign to the signs which are to be found in the rest of the body and which may serve to point to the cause – *guided observation, data gathering and hypothesis generation!*

Oedema

- Oedema is defined as an increase in the extra vascular/interstitial component of the extra-cellular fluid (ECF) volume.

'NORMAL' Oedema

- the obese
- the sedentary
- the gartered
- the corseted

Constriction of a limb leads to both venous and lymphatic obstruction and an increase in oedema.

Localised or Generalised

LOCAL OEDEMA may be due to inflammation, hypersensitivity or venous or lymphatic obstruction. GENERALISED OEDEMA usually has a systemic cause. When the cause is systemic the increase in ECF is of several litres before the oedema is obvious.

Acute swelling may be traumatic, inflammatory or related to venous thrombosis. By contrast *chronic* swelling of the limb or limbs may be caused by local venous or lymphatic block, a systemic cause or just be related to a sedentary lifestyle. Congestive cardiac failure will lead to an increase in venous pressure directly and, since the thoracic duct drains into the venous system, to an increase in lymphatic pressure as well as sodium and water retention by renal mechanisms.

Unilateral oedema usually has a local cause rather than a systemic one.
Bilateral oedema may be systemic in origin but a local factor such as dependency and chronic venous or lymphatic obstruction must be excluded.

Differential diagnosis

Is it oedema?

Remember to differentiate between an increase in volume due to fluid retention and one caused by an increase in bony or soft tissue.

327

Fluid distribution in the lower leg obeys Starling's hypothesis of capillary equilibrium between the arterial and venous ends of the capillary. Fine tuning of fluid flux depends on capillary permeability[1], plasma and interstitial fluid oncotic pressures and the interstitial fluid hydrostatic pressure which will be influenced in turn by posture and the calfmuscle pump effect on the lymphatic channels and veins.

FLUID *OUT* OF THE CAPILLARY
influenced by:

Mean intracapillary pressure[2] (**A**) +
Interstitial fluid oncotic pressure[3] (**B**)

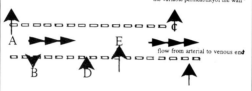

the variable permeability of the wall[4]

flow from arterial to venous end

direction of fluid flux

FLUID *IN* TO THE CAPILLARY
influenced by:

Mean interstitial liquid pressure[4] (**D**) +
Plasma oncotic pressure[5] (**E**)

---

[1]Changed by trauma or inflammation.
[2]Increased by cardiac failure or simple venous obstruction.
[3]The very high hydrostatic pressure in the feet means that the blood emerges at the venous end of the capillary with a consistency approaching treacle, and the excess fluid clearance from the tissues will rely greatly on the lymphatic channels aided by the calf muscle pump.
[4]Change may allow proteins to escape and lead to increased interstitial oncotic pressure.
[5]Dependent on the plasma proteins.

328

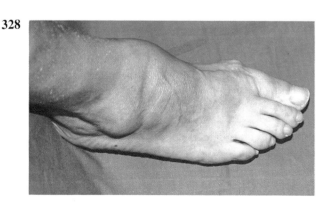

328 Fat pads at the ankle. The lateral side of the ankle, immediately anterior to the lateral malleolus overlying extensor digitorum brevis, is a common site for the laying down of fat. Often, the patient's complaint is of 'swollen ankles, Doctor!'. Fat pads do not pit, and can be differentiated from the muscle belly of extensor digitorum brevis which may be felt when the toes are retracted against resistance.

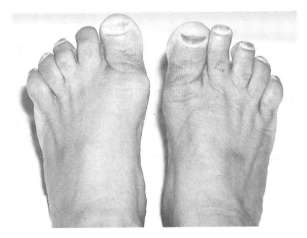

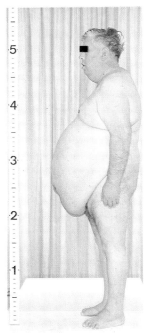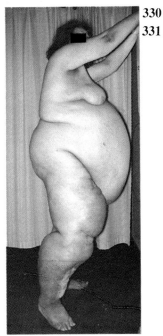

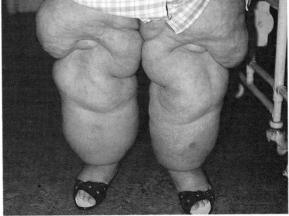

329 Soft-tissue increase in acromegaly. These female feet have enlarged over time, but the increase is in the soft tissues—redundant soft tissue over the dorsum of the foot. The toes are spatulate with bony tufting of the terminal phalanges. Henna was applied to the nails about four weeks ago.

330 Obese male. Pressure from the abdominal apron on venous and lymphatic channels increases the mean capillary pressure, which is further aggravated by a reduction in lymphatic flow due to inactivity and reduced calf pump action.

331 Obese female. The factors responsible for the oedema are unchanged, but are complicated by cellulitis, damage to lymph channels and a secondary lymphoedema.

332 and 333 Obese legs. The cause of the pitting oedema over the dorsum of the foot is mechanical pressure obstructing venous and lymphatic return.

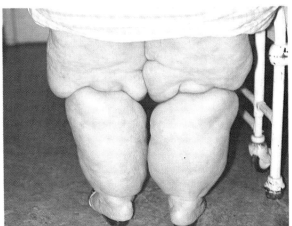

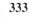

334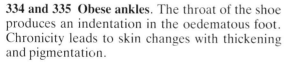

336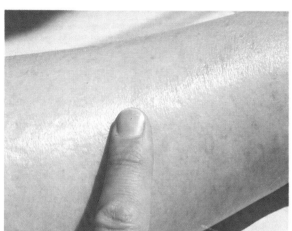

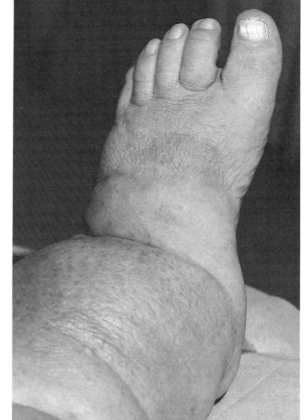

337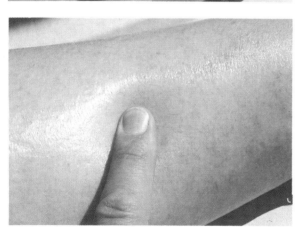

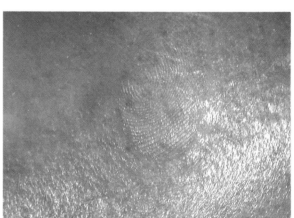

334 and 335 Obese ankles. The throat of the shoe produces an indentation in the oedematous foot. Chronicity leads to skin changes with thickening and pigmentation.

It is oedema!

336–338 Pitting oedema is the physical sign that the extravascular/interstitial proportion of the ECF is excessive. It is elicited by firm sustained pressure (**337**) on the surface; to show minor oedema, rather than a quick prod, it may have to be kept up for 15–20 seconds. When the digit is removed (**338**), a pit is left which may even show the fingerprint of the observer!

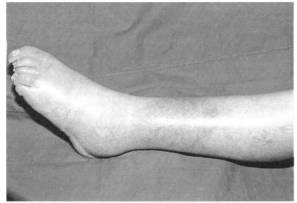

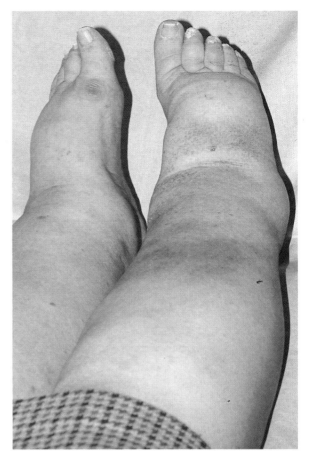

339 Oedema of the leg—congestive cardiac failure. Swollen, shiny and dependent oedema is often more easily elicited behind the malleolus by finger pressure when it is less obvious on the dorsum of the foot. A combination of increased mean capillary pressure, due to the increase in venous pressure, and secondary sodium and water retention by the kidney.

340 Oedema—congestive cardiac failure. The effect of gravity affects the distribution, the constrictive effect of the shoe prevents swelling of the toes, and there is erythema of shoe rub over the 1st metatarsophalangeal (mtp) joint. Chronicity leads to the brown pigmentation; the redness over the lower leg may be due to heat or recurrent thrombophlebitis.

341 Sacral pad: the effect of recumbency. Oedema may diminish on bedrest. This may be real and reflect a nocturnal diuresis, or it may simply reflect redistribution under the effect of gravity. If the sacrum is not examined, the physical sign of a pitting sacral pad of oedema will be missed.

For what reason?

The distribution of oedema gives an important clue to the cause. If it is confined to one limb, it is likely to be due to venous or lymphatic obstruction. In hypoproteinaemia, it will be generalised; it is likely to be evident in the lax tissues of the face and to be obvious on rising in the morning. By contrast, the oedema of heart failure tends to be present in the legs at the *end* of the day, and if the subject is confined to bed then the oedema will gravitate to the buttock and sacrum.

If it is bilateral then it is usually due to cardiac, hepatic, renal or nutritional conditions, and examination must aim to confirm or exclude them. Remember to assess the jugular venous pressure and to test the urine for albumen.

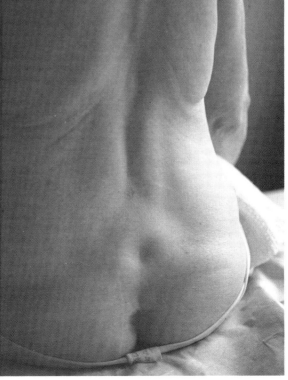

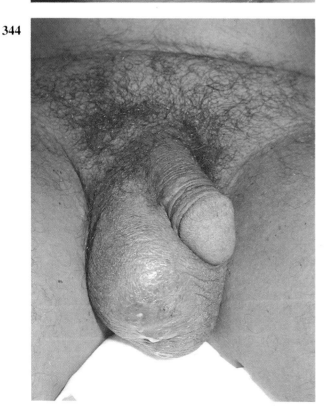

the variable permeabilityof the wall[4]

A

E

flow from arterial to venous end

B   D

direction of fluid flux

The permeability coefficient will change if the capillary wall becomes more permeable – for instance if damage or inflammation occurs.

342 If the permeability of the capillary changes, then fluid and proteins may leak into the interstitial space, as a result of trauma, inflammation, and the liberation of histamine and kinins. A change in permeability may account for the oedema in hypothyroidism and for the idiopathic oedema of women.

Inflammation due to infection

343 An infected ingrowing toe nail. *Rubor, calor, dolor, tumor*—red, hot, painful and swollen—these are the cardinal signs of inflammation. The cause of the swelling is usually obvious from its localisation and the associated history and signs; here, it is due to the migration of fluid in the inflammatory process.

344 Infected swollen scrotum. Oedema of the overlying skin and induration of the scrotal contents are due to a tuberculous epididymitis.

345 Acute erysipelas. This woman has a red oedematous foot showing pitting; the right foot has the scar of a Keller's operation overlying the 1st mtp joint. She presented with rigors followed by soreness in the groin; only later was some redness and tenderness noted on the foot. The redness spread over all of the dorsum and the groin glands became more tender. Rapid improvement occurred with penicillin—but not before a doctor had attempted treatment with a steroid cream, thinking the cause to be an allergy to leather![6]

343

1/1.2x

344

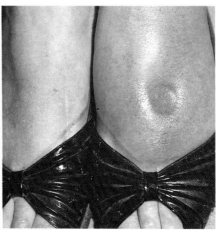

345

[6]*See* Chrome leather hypersensitivity.

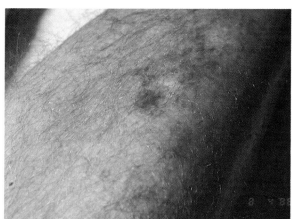

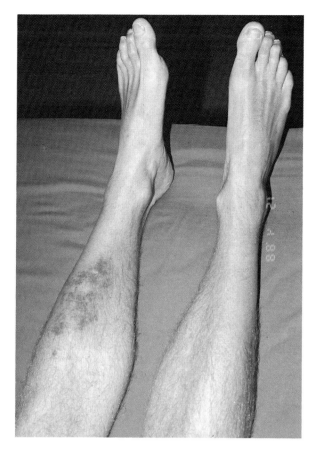

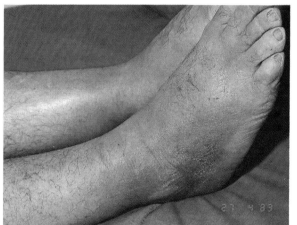

346 and 347 Erysipelas. The physician patient diagnosed the red patch (**346**) overlying the middle third of the left tibia initially as 'flu, then as a groin hernia, and finally—when the red hot tender area appeared on the leg—as erythema nodosum. The spreading red edge with oedema of the skin gradually subsides, and may fade, although the pitting oedema is still seen (**347**). The protein which seeps into the interstitial space may excite a chronic fibrotic reaction and may account for the tendency to recurrence at the same site.

348 A post-erysipelas foot. Recurrent attacks may lead to firm oedema, with tethering of the skin as a result of chronic fibrosis excited by the protein in the tissues, and to decreased lymph flow. The skin over the toes and leg becomes thickened and verrucous, and a fold of skin cannot be pinched up—Stemmer's sign.[7] This is characteristic of a lymphostatic disorder,[8] which is typified by excess protein, oedema, chronic inflammation and excess fibrosis.

[7]Foldi, M. 'Lymphoedema'. In: Foldi, M., Casley-Smith, J.R. (eds) *Lymphangiology*, 667–82. Stuttgart: Schattauer-Verlag, 1983.
[8]Mortimer, P., Regnard, C. Editorial. 'Lymphostatic disorders', *British Medical Journal*, **293**: 347–8, 9 August 1986.

349

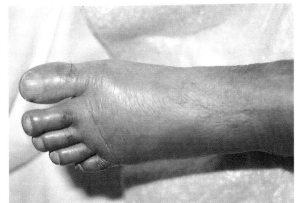

349 and 350 Diabetic synergistic gangrene. This diabetic has a swollen foot (**349**) from chronic infection and lymphostasis. On the heel (**350**), infection with aerobic and anaerobic organisms, producing a typical musty smell, has led to rapid tissue destruction.

350

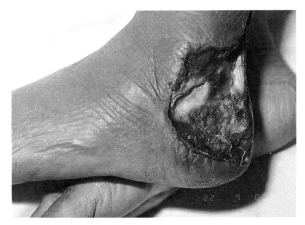

351

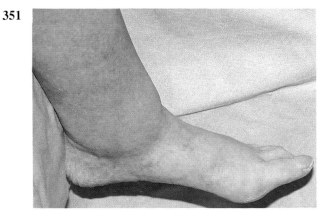

351 Cellulitis in a diabetic. The lower leg is tender, warm and swollen, with a demarcation line at the ankle.

352 Hypertrophic pulmonary osteoarthropathy (HPOA). Oedema of the ankle may overlie the periosteal reaction, best seen as a line of new bone formation on the tibia just above the medial malleoli. HPOA occurs with finger- and toe-nail clubbing and may reflect the increased vascularity; it may be associated with chronic inflammatory lung disease or carcinoma of the bronchus.

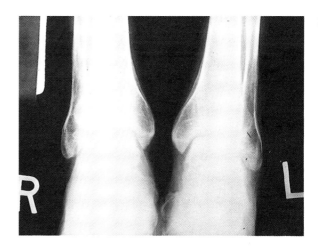

Inflammation of metabolic origin

353 A neuropathic subtalar joint, in a diabetic. The right ankle shows the dilated veins due to increased arteriovenous shunting of blood in an autonomic neuropathy. On the left, the ankle is swollen due to the development of a neuropathic subtalar joint precipitated by a relatively minor trauma (tripping at the pavement curb) and by the collapse of osteoporotic bone. The inflammatory reaction leads to swelling, but the joint continues to be used as little pain is felt.

353

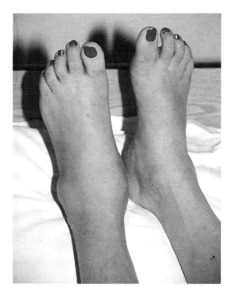

354 Acute gout podagra—presenting as acute inflammation of the 1st mtp joint, in a man who awoke during the night after his haemorrhoid operation with an exquisitely tender foot. The gout was precipitated by the man's long fast and the consequent ketosis.

354

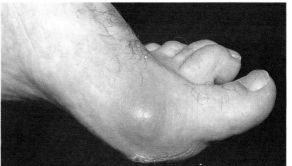

355

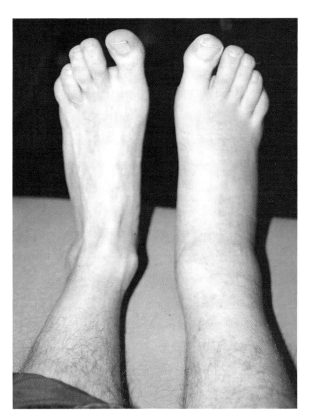

355 Midtarsal gout. By contrast with **354**, this man has marked swelling of the midtarsal area with much pain and pitting oedema. He had woken in the early hours with pain so bad, he thought he must have broken his foot, and so sought a radiologist the following day. The acute gout remained undiagnosed and untreated for 14 days.

356

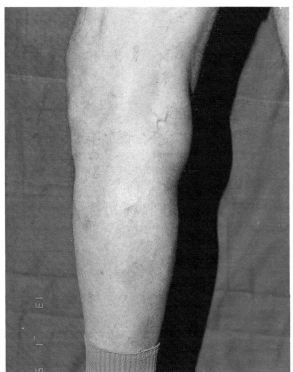

356 Popliteal, or Baker's* cyst.[9] The synovial swelling behind the knee which is thrown into prominence on extension may rupture, and the swelling produced may mimic a deep venous thrombosis or, if bilateral, be confused with a generalised cause for oedema.

*W.M. Baker (UK), 'On the formation of synovial cysts in the leg in connection with disease of the knee joint.' St. Bartholomew's Hospital report, **13**: 245–61, 1877.

Capillary leakage

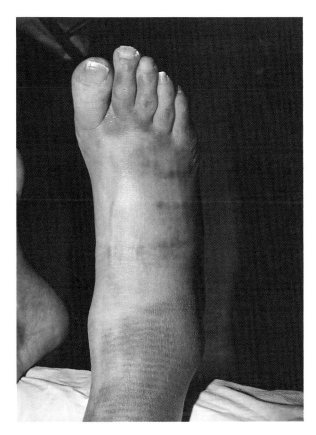

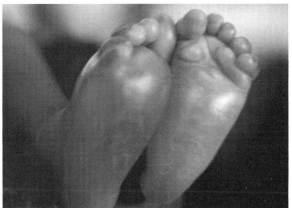

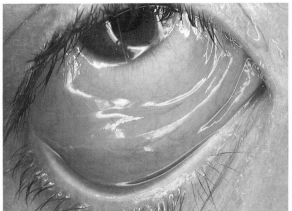

357 Oedema due to trauma. Capillary damage from physical trauma of a sprained ankle may lead to impressive swelling. Bruising may track a considerable distance.

358 Burnt feet. The thermal insult to feet immersed in a hot cooking pot leads to rapid exudation of fluid. In this West African child the burn may have been precipitated by loss of consciousness with a febrile convulsion resulting in a fall into the fire—or the convulsion may have been terminated by the child's immersion in the hot pot.

359 Chemosis of the conjunctiva. The eye has been rubbed with a finger contaminated by the pollen of a Venus fly trap plant, resulting in oedema of the conjunctiva. The substance created by this leads to the release of endogenous histamine, which changes the permeability of the capillary.

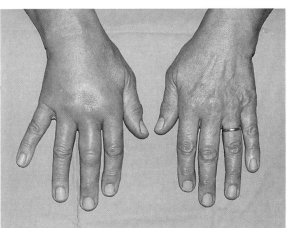

360 Insect bite hand. The injection of hymenoptera venom may produce a local erythema at the site, followed by liberation of histamine and oedema. A systemic anaphylactic reaction in a susceptible individual with an IgE reagin response may occur.

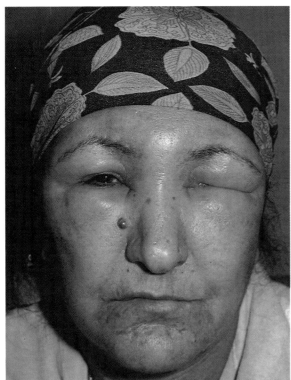

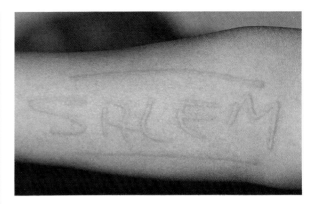

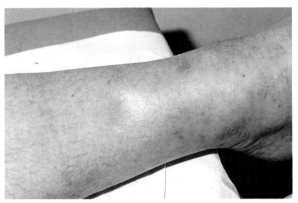

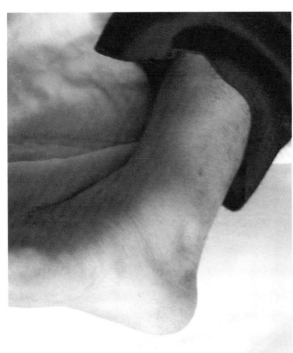

361 Angioedema face (penicillin allergy). This periorbital oedema occurs after parenteral penicillin therapy. It involves the skin and the deeper layers of the subcutaneous tissue. It may be IgE-dependent and due to a specific antigen sensitivity (**360 and 361**), complement-mediated as in hereditary angioedema and serum sickness, non-immunologic by direct mast-cell releasing agents like contrast media or aspirin and non-steroidal anti-inflammatory drugs (NSAIDS).

362 Dermographism. An exaggeration of the normal wheal and flare in response to scratching of the skin. The initial capillary blanching is followed by a reflex flare of vasodilatation and increased permeability following local histamine release.

363 Hypothyroidism. Firm pressure behind the medial malleolus must be used to show minor oedema. This man has severe hypothyroidism and his oedema cleared over the first month's replacement therapy. The oedema related to increased capillary wall permeability.

364 Oedema in diabetes—autonomic neuropathy. Increased blood flow, together with arteriovenous shunting, accompanies autonomic neuropathy in the limb. It is associated with oedema.

Venous blockage *increases* mean intra-capillary pressure

365 and 366 Acute superficial thrombophlebitis. A tender palpable vein with surrounding erythema, warmth and oedema. It gradually subsided over seven days and the overlying skin peeled (**366**). The condition is not associated with pulmonary embolism. Migrating superficial thrombophlebitis may be a marker of an underlying malignancy.

367 Acute deep venous thrombosis (dvt). The swelling of the left leg is a consequence of an increase in the mean capillary pressure. The blue tint in the same leg is due to cyanosis of the blood in the stagnant veins. Tenderness, where it occurs, reflects the size of the inflammatory reaction. A clot is propagated proximally and may break off and produce a pulmonary embolism.

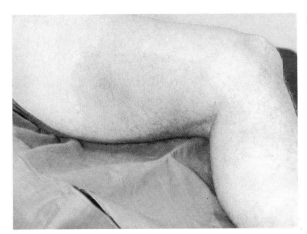
365

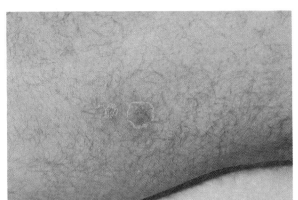
366

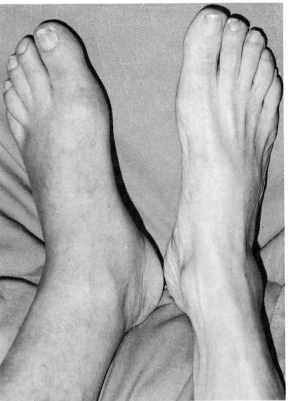
367

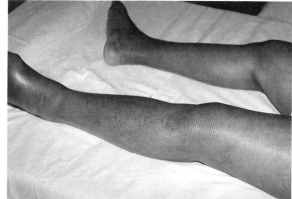

368 Deep venous thrombosis (associated carcinoma pancreas). More extensive oedema in a leg with proximal deep vein thrombosis with calf and thigh tenderness. Predisposing stasis, vascular damage and hypercoagulability are the factors common to the conditions in which venous thrombosis occurs: bedrest, surgery, trauma, malignant disease, and a spectrum of diseases associated with increased coagulability.

369 Residual venous dilation. Recanalisation may occur though residual obstruction in the deep venous system may be reflected in dilatation of the superficial veins in this man's left leg.

370 DVT residual old oedema. When the venous system is extensively blocked, severe residual swelling remains which the lymphatic channels cannot cope with, leading to chronic oedema due to venous insufficiency.

371 Varicose veins. Superficial, dilated and tortuous; a complication of incompetent valves so that the head of pressure is transmitted to the unsupported vein and to the capillary. Irritating varicose eczema and hyperpigmentation related to leakage and breakdown of red cells may develop, and be followed by ulceration about the malleoli.

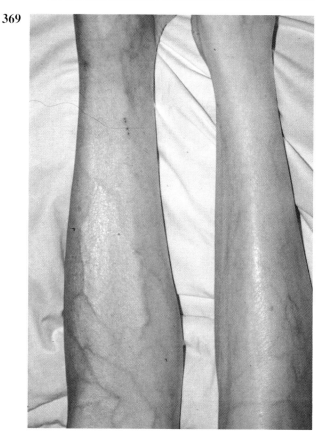

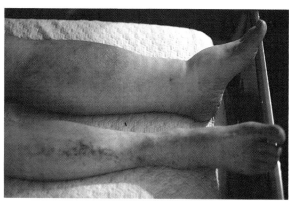

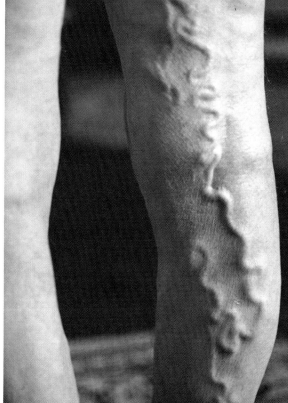

372 Chronic venous insufficiency. Oedema of the right leg due to increased mean capillary pressure. Leakage of protein leads to inflammation and fibrosis with secondary lymphoedema and verrucous change of the overlying skin. Ulceration is present above the lateral malleolus. There is a redness on the medial aspect of the leg—the lymphoedema predisposes to recurrent cellulitis.

373 and 374 Proximal venous blockage. A Cypriot seamstress complained of a swollen left leg (**373**). She operated a treadle sewing machine with her right foot for six days a week. No signs were found in the legs—the inexperienced physician explained that the inactive left leg did not utilise the calf pump to increase lymph and venous flow and thus led to sedentary unilateral oedema with an increase in mean capillary pressure! He was embarrassed to see a calcified pelvic fibroid on the X-ray (**374**) which was easily felt when a full examination of the patient was performed which included pelvic assessment. The mean capillary pressure was raised due to extrinsic pressure on the veins in the pelvis.

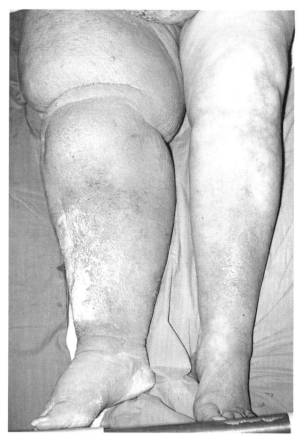

372

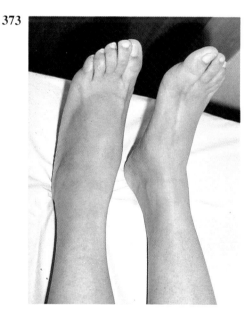

373

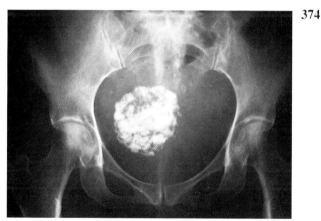

374

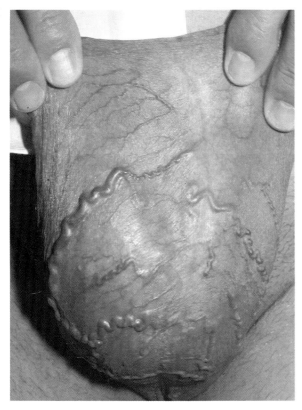

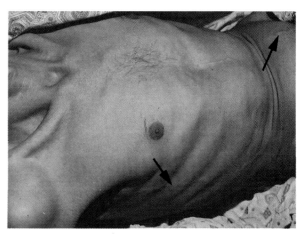

37

375 Oedema and varicosities of the scrotum. Block of the inferior vena cava (ivc) leads to a mean increase in capillary pressure, and an increase in fluid entering the extravascular interstitial space, which in turn leads to a compensatory increase in lymph flow. This man had moderate bilateral oedema and dilated superficial veins overlying the scrotum.

376 Prominent dilated veins on the abdomen (ivc block). The collateral venous system has developed over the abdominal wall to bypass the block. Veins can be seen coursing upwards in the epigastrium and over the lateral thoracic wall. The direction of flow is upwards.

Increase in mean capillary pressure

A central change in pressure in congestive cardiac failure will lead to peripheral oedema. The primary problem is an increase in venous pressure with a secondary consequence of renal under-perfusion leading to salt and water retention. The oedema of cardiac failure may be seen in the feet at the end of the day, but in the bedbound it may

gravitate to the dependent part of the body as a sacral pad. There may be evidence of cardiac failure with an elevated jugular venous pressure, a large liver with hepato-jugular reflux and a displaced apex beat reflecting cardiac enlargement as well as chest crackles heard on auscultation, indicating pulmonary fluid.

377 Oedematous feet with clubbed and cyanosed nails. These observations allow some deductions. The man is not anaemic—you need haemoglobin to be able to show cyanosis.[9] The oedema is bilateral, so the cause is most probably systemic rather than localised; pitting oedema is present over the dorsum of the foot. Cardiac, renal, hepatic and nutritional causes must be excluded. Nail clubbing and oedema with cyanosis suggest either a cardiac right-to-left shunt with cardiac failure and clubbing, or cor pulmonale from hypoxic lung disease and heart failure. . . . He has cryptogenic fibrosing alveolitis, cyanosis, clubbing and heart failure.

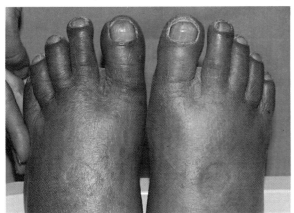

[9]An increase in reduced haemoglobin. In the Caucasian, it can be detected when the oxygen saturation is reduced to 85%, but in the dark-skinned it may not be apparent until oxygen sat. falls to 75%. Either there is an increase in the total venous blood in the skin or oxygen sat. falls. It can be seen when the mean capillary concentration of reduced Hb exceeds 5 g/l. The absolute value rather than the relative one is important. Thus, in anaemia one can have marked desaturation

and see no cyanosis, and in polycythaemia one may be cyanosed at higher levels of oxygen sat.

Central cyanosis: caused by arterial desaturation or abnormal haemoglobin.

Peripheral cyanosis: caused by slowing of flow and increased extraction of oxygen.

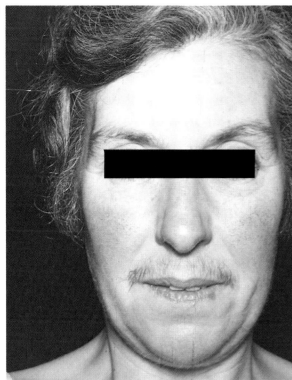

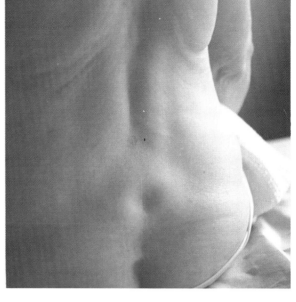

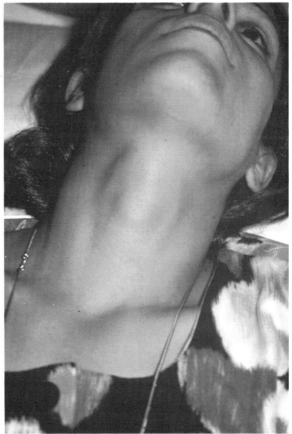

378 Mitral facies. There is a cyanotic flush over the malar areas—the malar flush. The face is pinched: this sign is seen in severe mitral stenosis and reflects peripheral vasoconstriction with reduction in cardiac output and increased extraction of oxygen during the slow passage of the blood through the skin. A central component relates to minimal arterial hypoxia due to secondary fibrotic changes in the lung consequent on long-standing congestion.

379 Sacral pad. Elevated mean capillary pressure leads to oedema, which may shift overnight to the dependent sacrum, disappearing from the ankles. The pitting can be elicited by sustained firm pressure.

380 Elevated internal jugular venous pressure (j.v.p.). The increase in right atrial pressure in cardiac failure is transmitted back to the valveless internal jugular vein. The engorged veins can be seen on either side of the larynx and pulsate with the transmitted pressure waves from the atrium. The venous pressure is high, the top of the venous column reaching the angle of the jaw when the patient is resting at 45 degrees to the horizontal. Observation of the pattern of wave form and the height of the column above the sternal angle give valuable information. The vertical height between the top of the column is usually less than three centimetres and the atrium lies about 5 cm below the angle = 8 cm of blood.

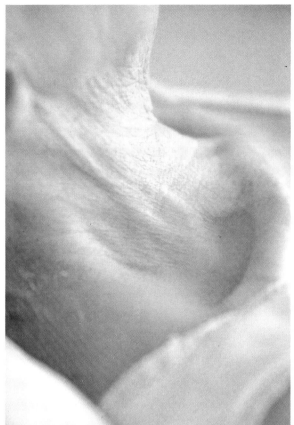

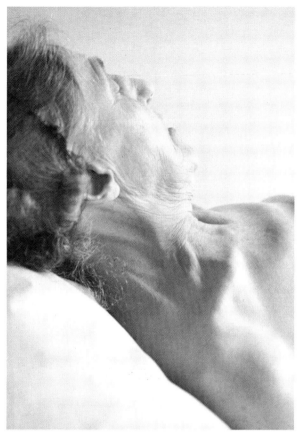

383

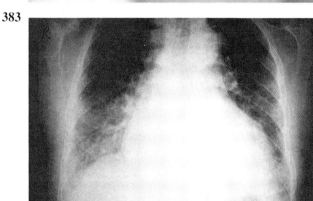

381 and 382 Elevated jvp external jugular before (381) and after (382) abdominal compression. Pitfalls to avoid in observing the venous pressure include measuring the height of the venous column in the external jugular vein, since the latter may be kinked and give a false impression of an elevated pressure: this problem will not arise if the internal jugular is used. If the liver is compressed by right upper abdominal pressure the venous column will rise and the free oscillations confirm direct communication with the atrium. Hepatojugular reflux of blood on compression is marked if the liver is engorged from an increased right atrial-filling pressure, and may be brought out if the patient breathes in during compression and thus enhances the venous return to the heart.

384

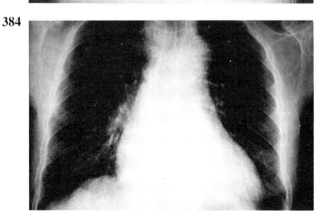

383 and 384 Chest X-ray of a big heart (**383**), in a case of **congestive cardiac failure**. The increased venous pressure is reflected in the pulmonary venous congestion of the lung fields, the apex beat displacement reflecting the cardiac enlargement due to dilatation of the chambers. The cardiac diameter is increased in comparison to the thoracic diameter, the cardiothoracic ratio being greater than 1:2. After diuretic therapy (**384**), the venous congestion has disappeared and the heart has become smaller.

385 and 386 Pallor. Severe anaemia leads to a high output state of the heart and may lead to heart failure. Anaemia may produce pallor of the palm (**385**, where it is contrasted with the examiner's) or of the conjunctiva (**386**, where it is compared with the nailbed)—though use of the latter site may lead to confusion, as it may be pale even when the subject is *not* anaemic. The tongue and buccal mucosa are less misleading.

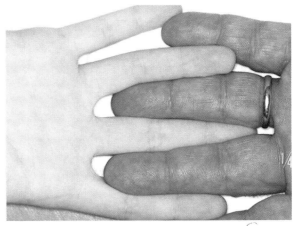

385

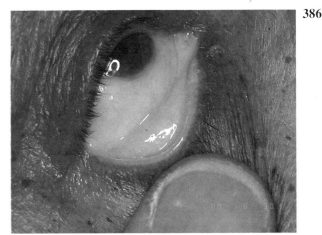

386

Increase in mean capillary pressure as a consequence of salt and water retention

387 Steroid facies. This teenager has generalised puffiness, due to a combination of fluid retention and steroid-induced obesity. His face is moon-shaped with blocked pores, acne, lank hair and greasy skin. There is facial plethora. The classic Cushingoid face of steroid excess.

An overall increase in the ECF will lead to oedema. Fluid retention due to salt and water retention may occur in endogenouos and exogenous corticosteroid excess, as well as that induced by drugs such as non-steroidal anti-inflammatory preparations and vasodilators such as nifedipine.

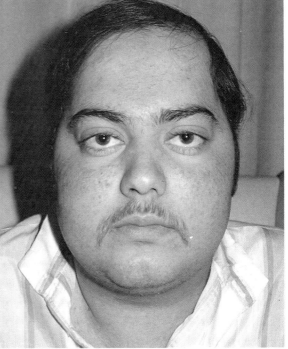

387

388

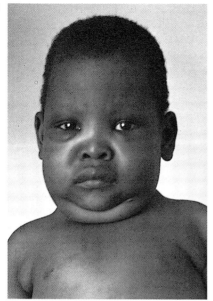

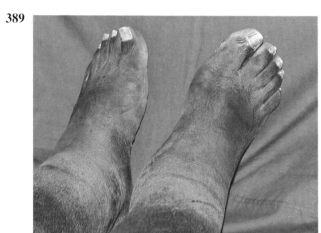

389

390

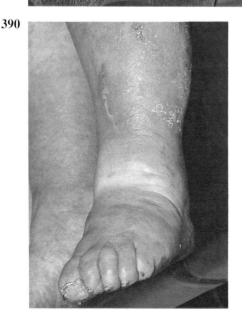

388 The nephritic facies of acute glomerulo-nephritis. Salt and water retention lead to oedema which is often more marked in the morning and is seen in the lax tissues of the face and periorbital areas. The clue to the cause may lie in testing the urine and finding blood and protein. This oedema is characteristically associated with haematuria, proteinuria and hypertension. Some of the oedema may be due to increased capillary permeability, but the major factor is salt and water retention by the kidneys due to renal insufficiency.

Fluid accumulation where increase in mean capillary pressure is aggravated by a reduction or block in lymph flow and/or a change in the interstitial fluid pressure or capillary permeability

Failure to use calf pump mechanism and the effect of gravity

389 The night security worker. This man sits in a booth near the factory exit throughout the night shift, and by the television set all day. Save for his journey to and from work he sits all the time, going to bed only on his night off! He has chronic puffy legs due to this sedentary life. The mean capillary venous pressure at the ankle means that the blood emerges with a relative treacle consistency. Freedom from oedema relies on activity and the calf pump mechanism massaging fluid up the lymph vessels, as well as facilitating the venous return. Drugs—including corticosteroids and non-steroidal anti-inflammatory agents, and carben-oxolone for gastric ulcers—may lead to fluid retention and oedema. Nifedepine and other dihydropyridine calcium antagonists may produce dependent oedema due to the impairment of the reflex increase in precapillary resistance that occurs when the legs are lowered and the hydro-static pressure in the capillary increases. Both pre-capillary permeability and blood flow may increase, and fluid leaks into the extravascular space.[10]

390 The sedentary alcoholic. The patient sold her bed to buy alcohol and so has to sit with the legs dependent on her remaining hard chair. These chronically oedematous legs have both reduced lymph flow and increased mean capillary pressure, forcing the equilibrium in the direction of fluid accumulation.

[10]Opie, L.H. 'Fluid retention with nifedepine in antihypertensive therapy.' *Lancet*, 1986; **2**: 1456.

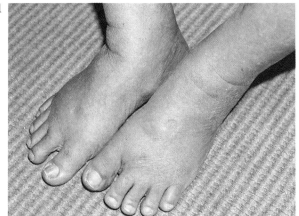

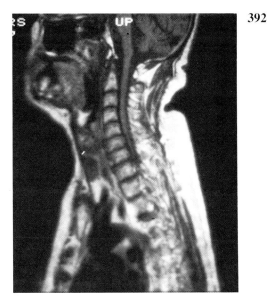

391–393 Paraplegic feet. The feet are puffy, and pitting oedema can be seen on the dorsum (**391**). The paraplegia is due to cervical cord compression leading to upper motor neurone paralysis of the legs, inactivity and oedema. The compression can be seen in the nuclear magnetic resonance scan (**392**) and the lower motor neurone wasting of the small muscles of the hand (**393**) in the guttering caused by the wasting of the 1st dorsal interosseus (T1 – ulnar) — a clue to the level of the lesion.

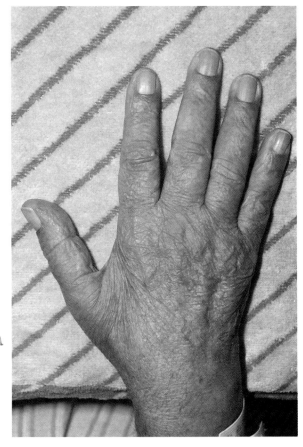

394

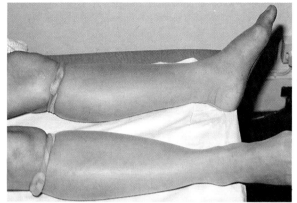

External compression and block of lymph and venous drainage

394 Tight garters and corsets. The complaint of oedema of the feet may have a prosaic cause. Garters may impair venous and lymphatic return, a fact which may not be appreciated by the patient.

395

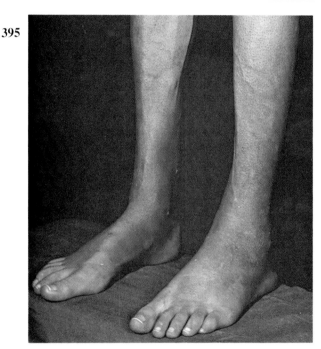

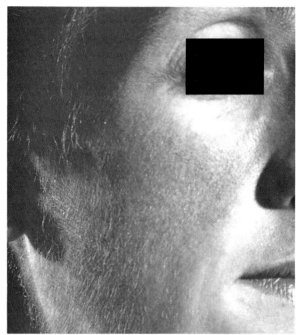

39

A change in oncotic pressure of the plasma

395 and 396 Legs, in a case of **anorexia nervosa**. The legs (**395**) are emaciated and may have a brown colour, the skin is dry and scaly, and lanugo hair is seen on the face (**396**). A morbid fear of being fat may lead to a radical restriction

Oedema due to hypoproteinaemia

inadequate intake

of food intake and consequent emaciation and weight loss. Oedema is infrequently a feature, and is due less to hypoproteinaemia than to a relative maintenance of the ECF compared with the loss of body mass.

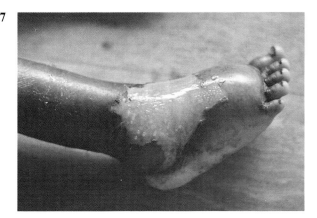

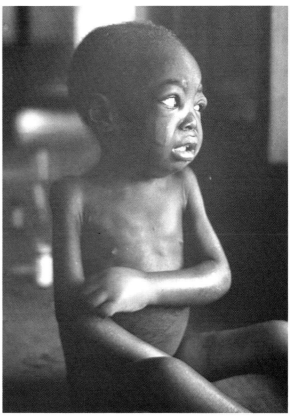

397 Legs, in a case of **protein/calorie malnutrition**. Contrasting with **395**, the leg of a child with protein/calorie malnutrition shows oedema related to a low plasma oncotic pressure, dry flaky skin which peels, and a characteristic craquelure* of malnutrition which may be appreciated in an individual with malabsorption due to small bowel disease (**401–403**).

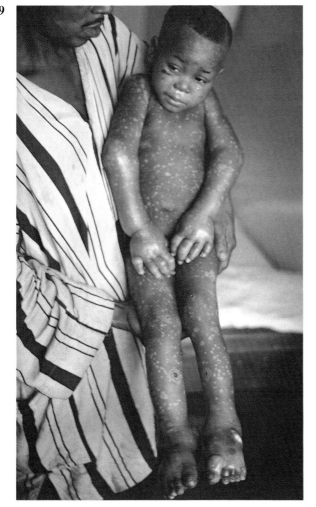

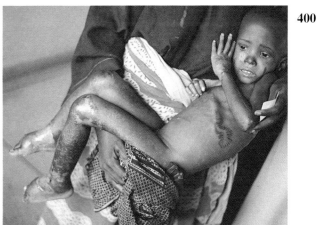

398–400 Child facies and posture. Kwashiorkor—protein/energy malnutrition. Signs include a miserable demeanour, thin depigmented hair, anaemia, the pot belly, angular stomatitis and oedema—the latter related in part to hypoproteinaemia and in part to salt and water excess.

This syndrome may occur when there is insufficient energy to cover the body needs. Inadequate intake, increased demands following disease (such as measles—**399**), and bodily losses after gastroenteritis (**400**): may all produce a similar picture.

*A network of small cracks in the paint or varnish of the surface of a painting.

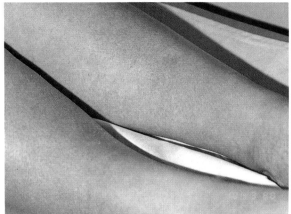

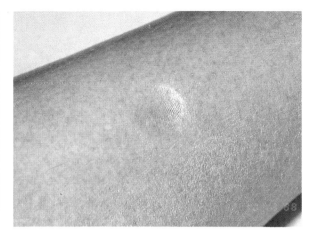

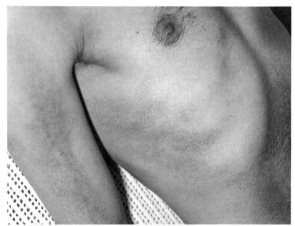

Malabsorption

401–405 Minimal oedema and skin change of the legs. The characteristic reticulate pigmentation and oedema (**402**) may be the presenting sign, and the pigmentation may be seen on other parts of the skin (**403**).

This man had a history of diarrhoea, whose greasy stools (**405**) had proved difficult to flush down the toilet. These fat-laden steatorrhoeal stools were in fact produced by the widened small bowel loops of small intestinal disease—small bowel lymphoma—visible in **404**.

Liver disease

This may be suggested by ascites, by collateral vessels, jaundice, or spider naevi. The ascites and increased intra-abdominal pressure may also obstruct the venous return from the lower limbs and further aggravate the oedema.

404

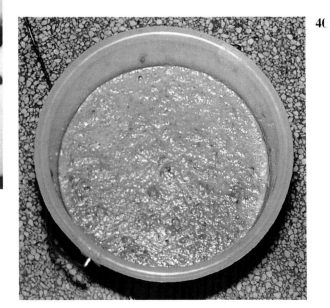

Signs which point to the liver as the cause of the oedema

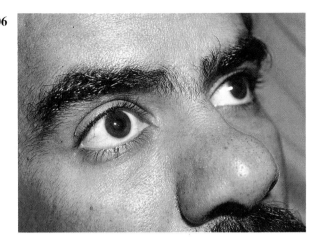

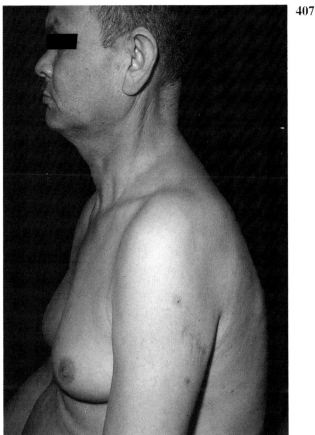

406 The jaundiced eye. Very slight jaundice may be reflected in a lemon tint of the sclera. Jaundice may be due to obstruction to the outflow of bile, to hepatocellular dysfunction, or to haemolysis.

407 Gynaecomastia. The enlarged breasts and arterial spider angiomas seen on the arm are both due to chronic liver disease. Breast enlargement is related to disturbance in hormonal metabolism, although spironolactone—an aldosterone antagonist—given as a diuretic, may lead to breast enlargement.

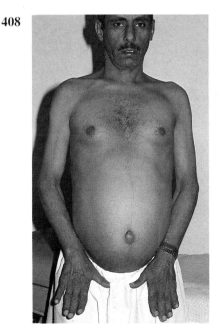

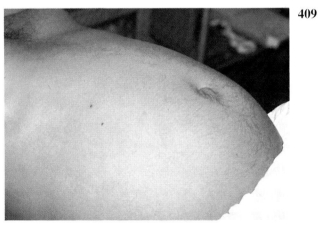

408 and 409 Ascites. The eyes show yellow sclerae, indicating jaundice. The belly is distended, and there is an umbilical hernia which is full of ascitic fluid and empties when the man lays down (**409**). The nail tips are buffed and glossy from his scratching. Gynaecomastia is present. The low albumen is a factor in the production of ascites.

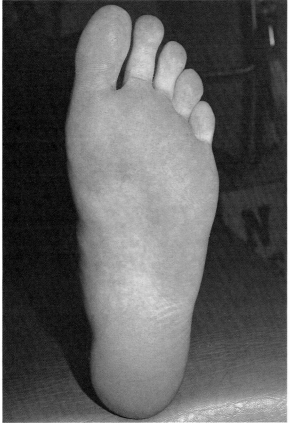

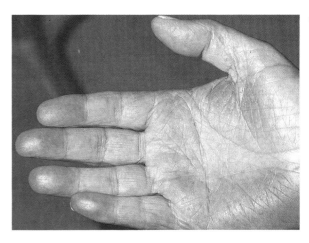

410 and 411 Erythema: liver soles and liver palms. Palmar and plantar erythema may be a feature of liver disease, but it is also seen in pregnancy and thyrotoxicosis. It should not be confused with erythromeialgia.[11] This condition may be associated with thrombocythaemia and relieved by aspirin. Primary erythermalgia is first seen in childhood; it is bilateral and symmetrical, and aggravated by exercise and warmth. Secondary erythermalgia is seen in gout, and in collagen disease as Systemic Lupus Erythematosus and Polyarteritis Nodosa unassociated with any platelet dysfunction.

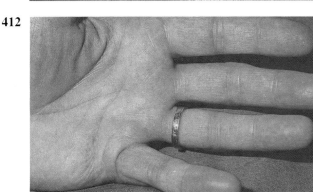

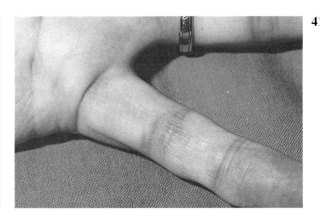

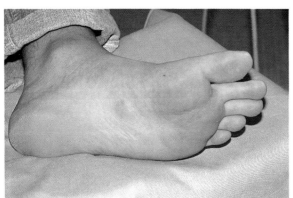

412–414 Dupuytren's contracture: sole and hand. This deformity produced by fibrosis of the palmar fascia results in flexion contracture of the fingers. It is felt first as a nodularity in the palm and seen as puckering of the skin (**412**). It is associated with alcoholism rather than cirrhosis, and may occur in users of vibrating tools, in cases of diabetes and diabetic retinopathy, and epilepsy. In the Dupuytren's nodule of the plantar fascia (**414**), contractures do not occur; the nodules are not painful but may be multiple.

[11]Editorial, *British Medical Journal*, **301**: 454–5, 1991.

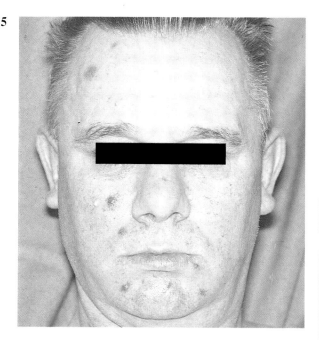

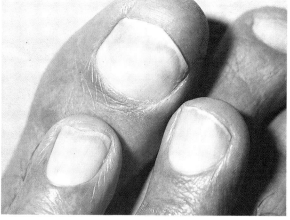

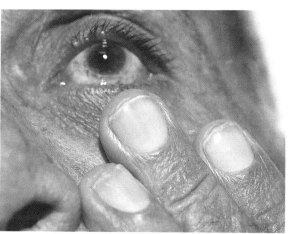

415 Facies with multiple arterial spider angiomata. There is a central feeding arteriole which, if compressed, will lead to blanching of the lesion and a characteristic filling of the capillary halo on release. Spiders are associated with liver disease, but also occur in pregnancy and disappear within hours of delivery.

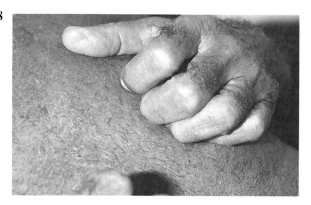

416–422 Shiny finger nails and dull toe nails. The tips of the finger nails may develop a marked polish from the friction of chronic pruritus and contrast with the dull tips of the toe nails. Compare this with the shiny toe nails that occur in children in cases of sock rub/stretch baby garments (see **81**). Buffed finger nail tips indicate a chronic itch, for which an explanation must exist. This man was complaining of puffy ankles, and had a tint of jaundice and highly polished nail tips (**417**). The liver function tests confirmed a cholestatic jaundice. In the act of scratching, tangential friction of the tips can be seen (**418**). If the complete nail is glossy, it has clear nail lacquer on it and the gloss will extend all the way to the cuticle (**419**). Itching may lead to excoriations, which may become pigmented and, typically, affect only the part that the patient can reach (**420**). In cholestasis, the urine may contain bile and the stools may be pale for lack of it. The dark bile-stained urine is on the right in **421**, next to a normal control.

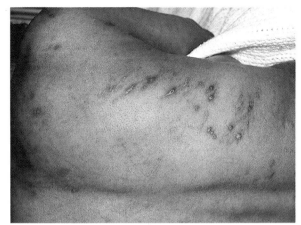

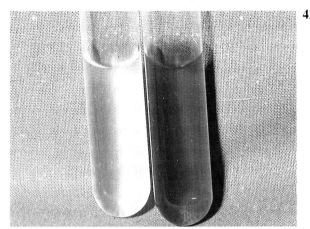

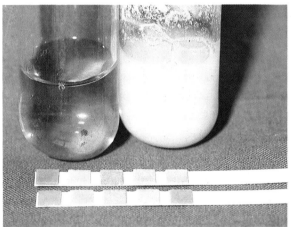

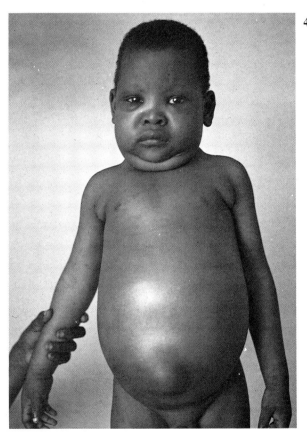

Loss of protein in urine or stool may lead to hypoproteinaemia

422 Heavy proteinuria before (left) and after (right) coagulation by boiling. Dipstick testing shows the presence of blood and protein. Individual squares from right to left in slide: pH, protein (+ + +), sugar (+), ketones (0), and blood (+).

423 A nephritic child. Gross proteinuria may lead to the nephritic syndrome. There is a puffy nephrotic facies as well as ascites.

Reduction in lymphatic flow

Chronic lymphatic obstruction may be associated with a change in the oncotic pressure of the interstitial fluid as well as to leakage of macromolecules.

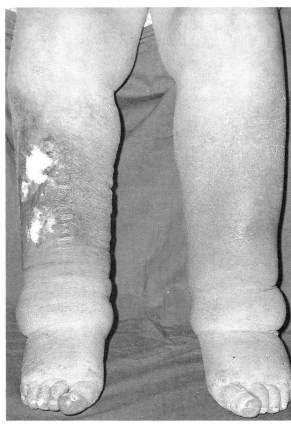

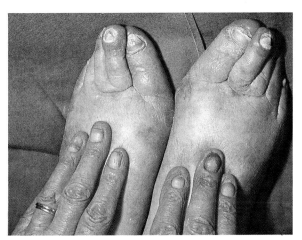

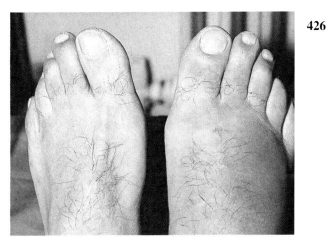

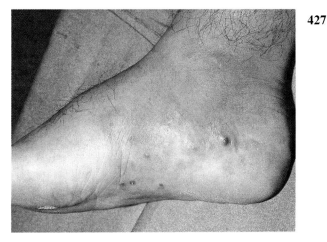

424 Congenital lymphoedema (Milroy's lymph-oedema).[12] Inadequate lymph vessels lead to chronic oedema with fibrosis, complicated by cellulitis and ulceration. The tissues are thickened and verrucous.

425 Yellow nail syndrome. There is oedema of the feet; the nails are thickened and vary in colour from yellow through to green, are slow growing, and may be shed—though, remarkably, they may also regrow.[13] The cuticle is absent. The lymphatic channels are sparse. Chronic lung disease—either pleural effusions or bronchiectasis—may be associated.[14]

426 and 427 Kaposi's sarcoma (HIV-negative) and oedema.[15] The form of Kaposi's sarcoma that is unassociated with HIV infection is seen in old age and frequently affects the extremities. Oedema is seen in association, and may reflect lymphatic obstruction. The raised purplish nodules are present on the plantar surface of the oedematous foot.

[12]Milroy, William Forsyth (1855–1942). 'An undescribed variety of hereditary oedema.' *N.Y. Med. J.,* **56**: 505–8, 1892.
[13]Samman, Peter D., White, W.F. 'The yellow nail syndrome.' *Brit. J. Derm.,* **76**: 53, 1964.

[14]Emerson, Peter. 'Yellow nails, lymphoedema and pleural effusions.' 1966.
[15]Kaposi, M. 'Idiopathisches multiple pigmentsarkam der Haut.' *Arch. Derm. Syph.* (Berlin) **4**: 265–73, 1872.

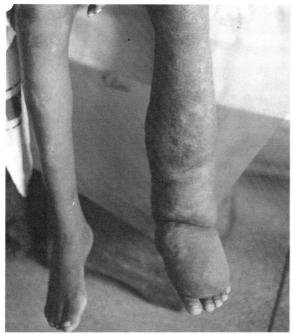

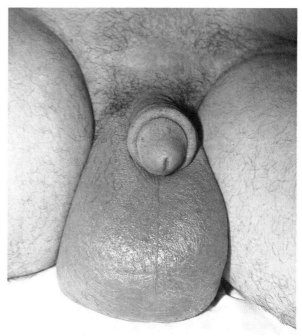

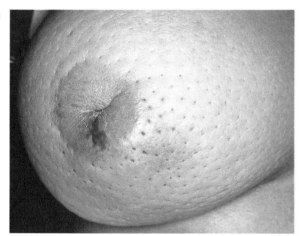

428 Filariasis oedema. Blockage of the lymphatics by the adult filarial parasites, where they reproduce sexually to yield large numbers of microfilariae which may appear in the blood, may lead to lymphoedema with thickening and brawny oedema.

Podoconiosis—non-filarial elephantiasis—is a disease of barefoot people, which begins in the teens with an area of erythema and burning, followed by persistent distal swelling of the foot and intermittent acute flares of discomfort. It is caused by penetration of the dermis by silica or aluminosilicates, which leads to lymphatic obstruction. Prevention is by wearing shoes.[16]

429 Oedema of the scrotum (carcinoma of the rectum). This man had an adenocarcinoma of the rectum with local spread. The blockage of the lymphatics leads to local oedema of the scrotum.

430 Oedema of the breast (*peau d'orange*). A reflection of tense dermal oedema due to tumour infiltration, but can arise in other circumstances when the superficial lymphatic plexus of the dermis is obstructed.[17]

[16]Price, E.W. 'Podoconiosis—non-filarial elephantiasis.' O.U.P. 1990.
[17]Mortimer and Ryan, *Lancet*, March 22, 1986.

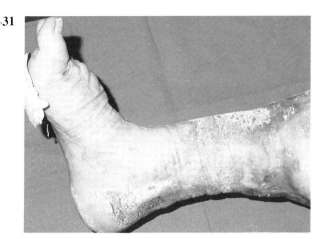

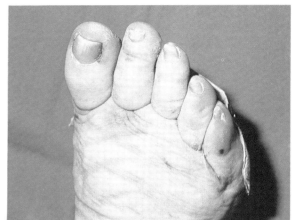

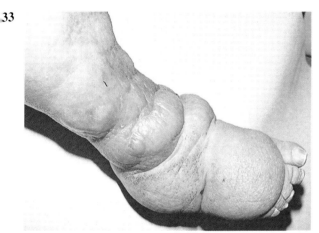

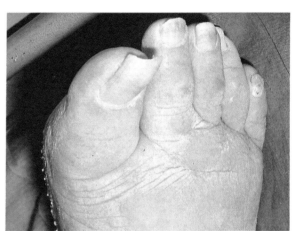

431–434 A healed gravitational ulcer and secondary lymphoedema. If normal lymphatics cannot keep pace with demand, and since their function is to remove protein and other macromolecules from the tissues, oedema associated with lymph stasis will have a high protein and macromolecule content which further withholds fluid osmotically, and also incites chronic inflammation and fibrosis: the pathology of lymphoedema. Thus, the skin becomes thickened and tethered (Mortimer *et al.*, *Lancet*, March 22, 1986), and later hyperkeratotic and verrucous—lymphoedema verrucosa. Pitting will occur but the tissues have a stolid feel.

9 The foot and endocrinology

As in the last chapter, the aim remains to lead the student from the foot, with its physical sign, to the signs found in the rest of the body. Changes seen in the foot caused by abnormalities of the endocrine system range from an increase in sweating, as in thyrotoxicosis and acromegaly, to the neglected foot which may hide the apathetic disinterest of hypothyroidism. Less mundane changes such as an increase in soft tissue in growth hormone excess are capped by the drama of gross pre-tibial myxoedema in thyroid acropachyderma. Even a dry foot may be a pointer to hypothyroidism or suggest the autonomic neuropathy of diabetes; oedema may reflect salt and water retention, or the thighs demonstrate livid striae if there is an excess of corticosteroids.

Pituitary gland

435

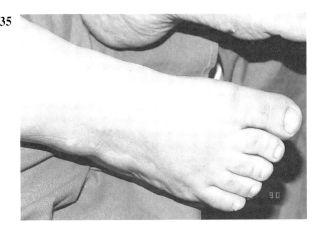

437

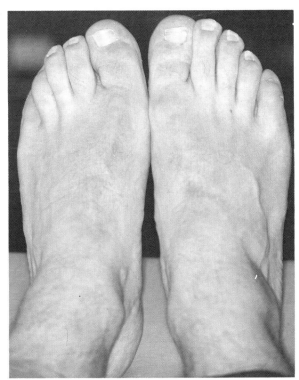

436

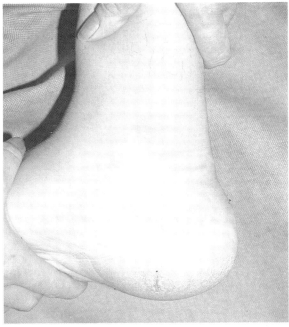

Excess growth hormone

435 Acromegaly: big feet. An increase in hand, foot and hat size may occur. A broad spade-like foot is typical, as there is an increase in soft tissue. Vitiligo, present laterally near the ankle joint, may be a pointer to other endocrine diseases, or to a multiple endocrine syndrome.

436 Acromegaly: prominent heels. There is an increase in the heel pad which sticks out of the line of the plantar surface.

437 Acromegaly: increased soft tissue on the dorsum of the feet. The increased soft tissue may be felt as redundant folds which can be picked up and spill into the interdigital spaces particularly seen between the first and second toes.

438

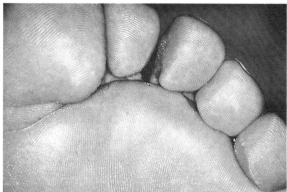

43

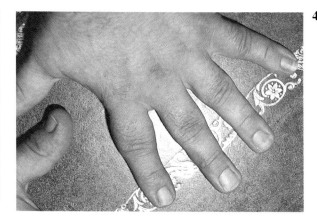

440

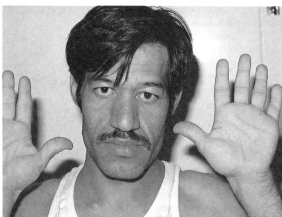

438 Acromegaly: the plantar aspect of the toes. Soft tissue bulges into interdigital spaces.

439 and 440 Acromegaly: spatulate hands (one male and one female). The fingers are broadened and spade-like from increased growth of the soft tissues. The nail folds rise up from the nail plates like earthworks, spilling back onto them. The cigarette burn overlying the distal interphalangeal (IP) joint of the middle finger (**440**) may be innocuous but it is a familiar sign in those prone to falling asleep while smoking, possibly under the influence of alcohol or drugs.

441

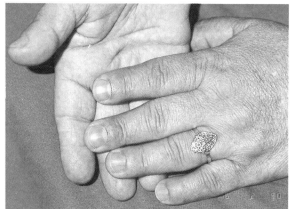

4

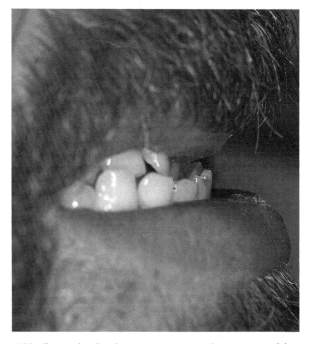

441 Acromegaly: facies and hands. In the palms of these typical acromegalic hands there is no thenar wasting, though median nerve compression due to tissue overgrowth in the carpal tunnel may occur. The glabellar ridges above the eyebrows are very marked and the soft tissues of the nose and lips are thickened and coarsen the facies. The mandible protrudes due to its overgrowth and produces an overbite.

442 (lateral view) **Acromegaly**: the prognathic jaw. The overbite of the incisors with the lower closing in front of the upper teeth are partly disguised by the full beard which this man has grown as a cosmetic distraction.

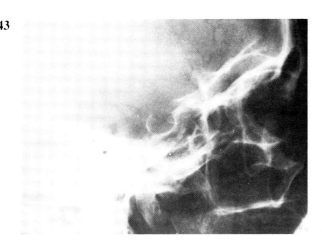

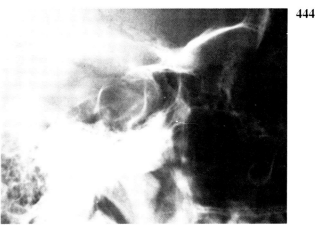

443 and 444 Lateral skull X-rays, comparing a normal pituitary fossa (**443**) with a ballooned pituitary fossa (**444**). The excess of growth hormone is produced by an adenoma of the pituitary —whose expansion may jeopardise adjacent endocrine cells, erode the bony walls of the fossa, and encroach on the adjacent optic chiasm.

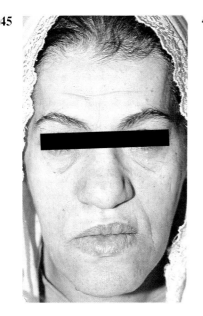

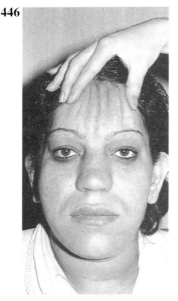

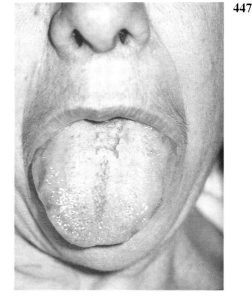
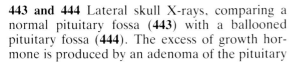

445–447 Acromegaly: facies. The face has little glabellar prominence, although the tissues of the nose are broadened and the jaw is prognathic (**445**). Over the forehead the redundant skin is thrown into relief and can be contrasted with your own (**446**)! Even the tongue may enlarge: remember that, if the tongue touches the angles of the mouth on protrusion, this may be due either to a small mouth *or* to a big tongue; the latter will demand consideration of hypothyroidism, acromegaly, primary amyloid, Down's syndrome, tumour, etc. (**447**).

Thyroid

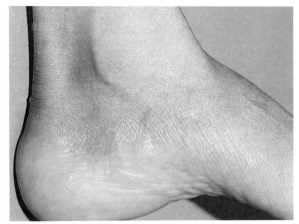

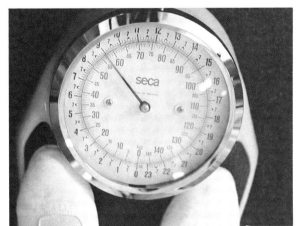

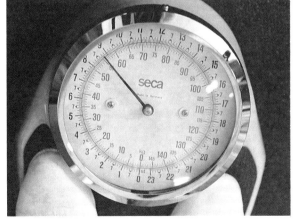

Overactive — thyrotoxicosis

448 Sweaty foot. An increase in the metabolic rate of thyrotoxicosis and acromegaly may make the individual sticky; where it leads to overt sweating, it may prompt a search for other signs. Sweaty feet occur commonly in youth, with exercise, in hot temperatures, or with fever and infection. Increased sympathetic activity from emotion, anxiety, hypoglycaemia or phaeochromocytoma may present with sweating. Sweating with eating may be stimulated by spices and alcohol, or occur in diabetes mellitus. Malignant disease such as lymphoma and leukaemia may present with recurrent sweats.

449 and 450 Weighing scales sign. Clinical assessment includes body weight: infrequently the pointer of a spring balance will not be still, and oscillates (**449**). In the thyrotoxic it reflects a combination of tremor and the recoil of the cardiac high output state. This is compared with a second reading (**450**), taken some weeks later, when the patient is euthyroid: now, the scales pointer is sharply focussed, and records a small weight loss!

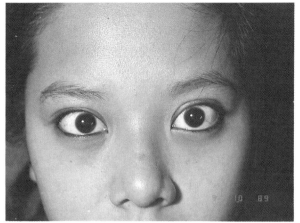

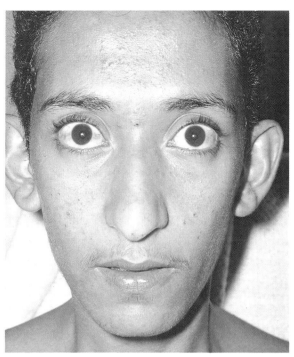

451–455 Lid retraction in, respectively, a Vietnamese, an Arab, and a European—the latter first *with* glasses, then without. The Vietnamese girl (**451**) complains of palpitations and has lid retraction of the right eye with a clear rim of sclera. The Arab boy (**452**) has bilateral lid retraction. The European (**453**) *looks* normal, but admits to feeling tense and sweaty—even though the weather is cold. He stood on the scales to be weighed and the pointer oscillated and failed to settle. When his glasses are removed (**454**), the proptosis of the right eye can be appreciated. After treatment, he gained weight and the eye signs are barely discernible (**455**).

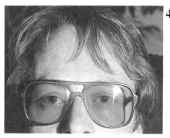

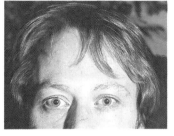

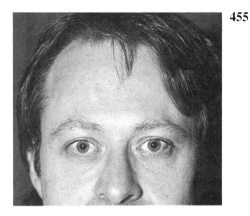

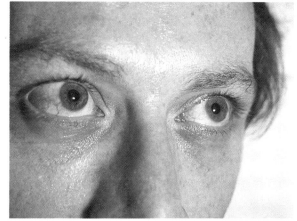

456

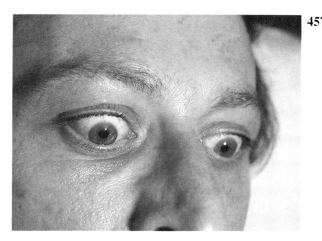

457

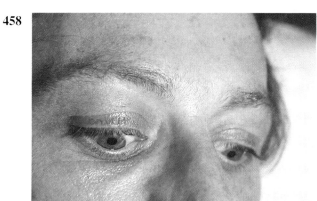

458

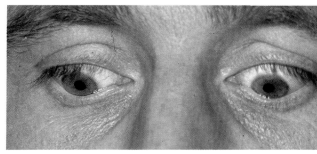

459

456–459 Lid lag. Lid retraction is due to increased activity of the levators of the eyelid. It may be emphasised by the protrusion of the eye—proptosis caused by an increase in orbital volume. The increase in levator palpebrae superioris activity leads to the phenomenon of lid lag: the lid fails to follow the eyeball downwards as the gaze is moved from the ceiling (**456**) to the floor with the head stationary, and a chink of sclera becomes visible (**457**) for a moment at the end of the movement, before the lid catches up with the eyeball (**458**). Though this man has no other eye signs—lid retraction, proptosis, periorbital oedema, chemosis, or external ocular palsy, for example— he looks hot, sweaty and thyrotoxic. Lid lag may occur if there is an abnormality of muscle tone (**459**) when the eye looks down after a period of protracted upward gaze. Here, the patient, being euthyroid, is clearly cool and dry skinned, but he suffers from myotonia congenita, with failure of rapid relaxation of the muscles at the end of sustained movement.

Lid retraction

460–463 Lid retraction: a spectrum. Lid retraction and slight (**460**), marked (**461**), and congested (**462**) proptosis of the right eye in thyroid eye disease. The woman complained that the right eyelid drooped! If the experience of the normal is small this confusion between the normal and abnormal side is an easy error. In **462** there is periorbital oedema, injection and chemosis of the conjunctiva which bulges, as well as lid retraction and proptosis disguised by the redness of the sclera. In **463**, the eye cannot close and has dried at the inner canthus . . . early malign exophthalmos. The subject, a chauffeur, became excessively agitated in traffic jams, and was referred by his employer.

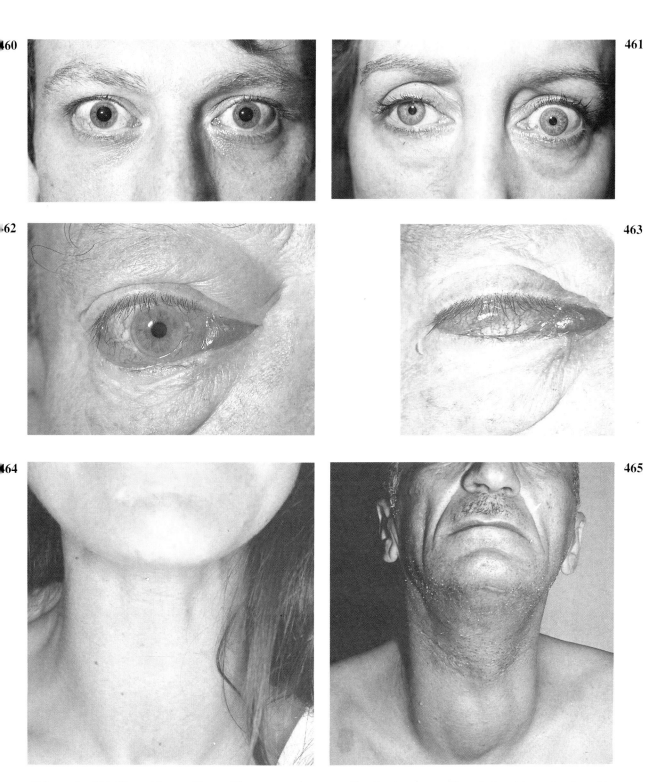

464 and 465 Thyroid swelling. The smooth symmetrical fullness of a simple goitre (**464**) is overlain by the sternomastoid muscles on either side and just intrudes into the suprasternal notch. It is best seen if the lighting is oblique. It is confirmed when the gland is seen to move on swallowing because of its relationship to the thyroid cartilage. The different shape of the goitre (**465**) is due to the presence of asymmetric nodules. The lateral lobes are visible bulging between the strap muscles of the neck.

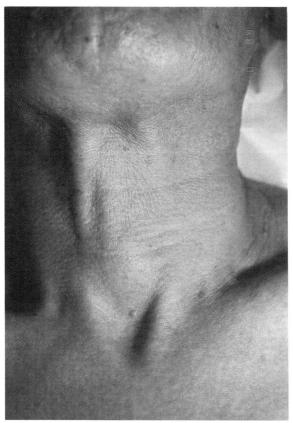

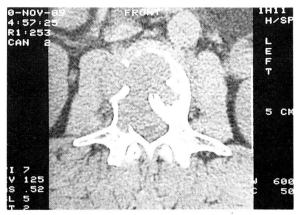

466 and 467 Thyroid nodule. A small thyroid nodule may be noticed bobbing about as the patient speaks or swallows. This man complained of sciatic pain, exacerbated by bending or coughing. As the leg was examined and muscular strength assessed, a glance upwards disclosed the small nodule which had just moved up from the sternal notch as the patient swallowed! It was a medullary carcinoma of the thyroid, and the pain was due to a deposit in the lumbar vertebra (**467**). The destruction of the body of the vertebra can be seen on the CAT scan.

468

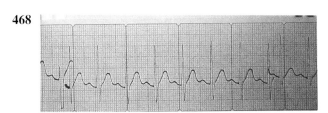

469

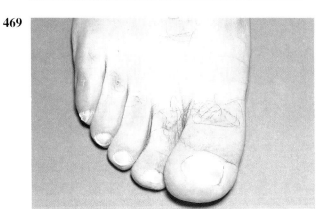

468 Palpitations. 'My heart beats so fast!' is the commonly heard refrain—and, indeed, the heart beat *does* increase during palpitations. The ECG trace (**468**) to show sinus tachycardia recorded 104 bpm after a 20-minute rest—when all signs of nervousness at being on the couch should have subsided, and with them the tachycardia! Tachycardia leads to a cardiac high-output state and may lead to cardiac failure. Auricular fibrillation may be the overt presentation of the occult over-active gland.

469–475 A pre-tibial myxoedema series over 15 years. This series shows a manifestation of thyroid auto-immune disease which affects the skin of the foot or leg, though rarely produces such gross changes with an increase in the volume of the foot. An increase in shoe size in thyroid disease may reflect oedema and cardiac failure. Six months after radio-active iodine for thyrotoxicosis, the skin has thickened and developed a characteristic pink colour over the great toes (**469–471**). During a ten-year period, in spite of heroic therapy, the changes progressed (**472 and 473**) and finger nail clubbing developed—thyroid acropachy (**474**). Proptosis and bilateral tarsorrhapies (**475**) can be seen.

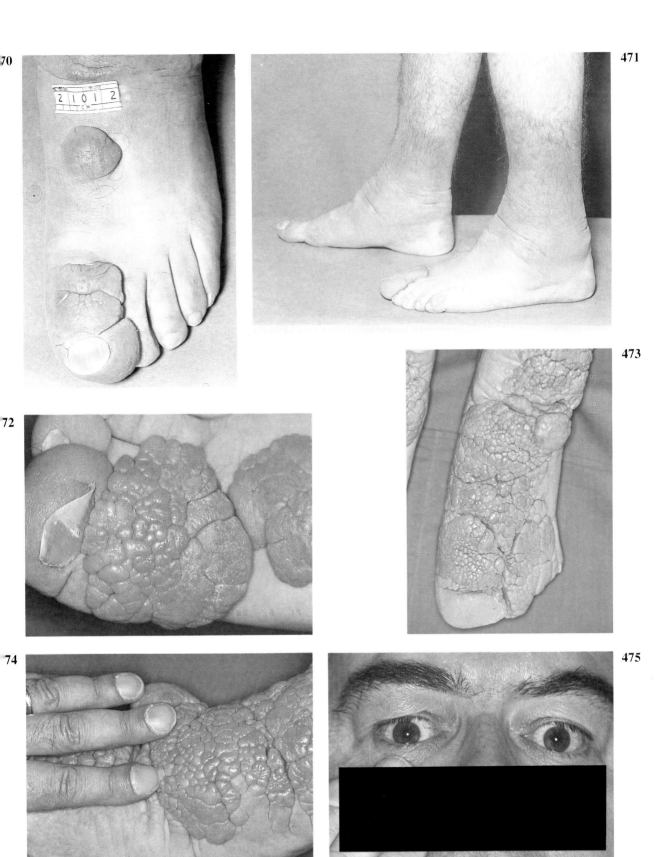

141

Thyroid

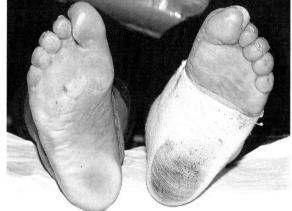

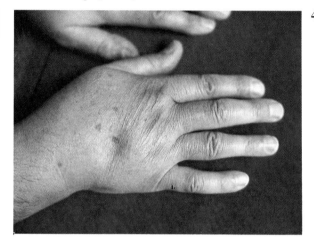

Hypothyroid/underactive

476 Neglected feet. A prosaic sign—the apathy of myxoedema is one reason why an elderly person may neglect the feet. There is always a reason for neglect, and if that isn't appreciated the chance to alleviate the underlying cause is lost.

Differential diagnosis on the medical significance of neglected feet:

mental—dementia, depression; psychosis
social—economic, housing, support, bereavement
medical—hypothyroid, diabetic, self-neglect, dm cataract
    —retinopathy → blind, partially sighted glaucoma
    —physically disabled, alcoholic.

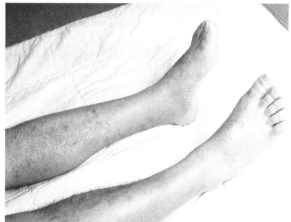

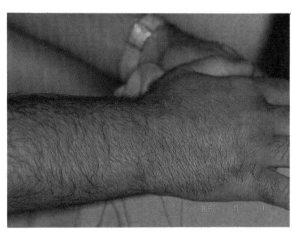

477–479 Oedematous feet—hypothyroid. The feet in **477** show oedema that pits on firm pressure. The body hair in both **477** and **478** is sparse and short, like mown stubble. This regrows after six months' thyroxine therapy, as **479** illustrates. The swelling, too, disappears.

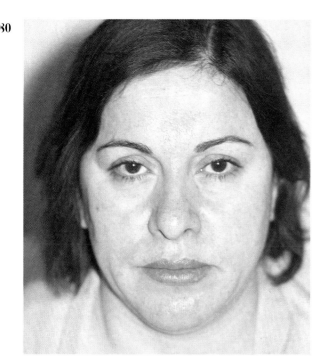

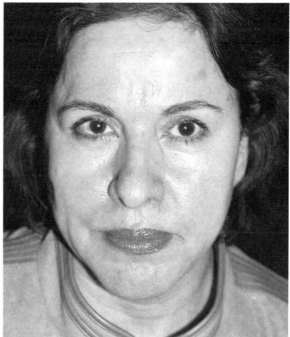

480 and 481 Facies of myxoedema before and after treatment. The face in the first illustration may be thought of as normal at a cursory glance. However, the possibility of hypothyroidism is usually appreciated following recognition of some symptom or sign. This woman has (in **480**) the characteristic fat face and stolidity of the condition—as becomes clearer when the *before* view is compared with that *after* treatment (**481**).

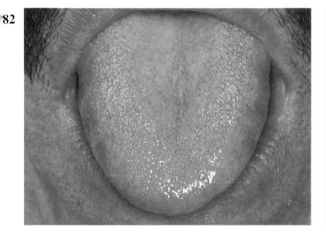

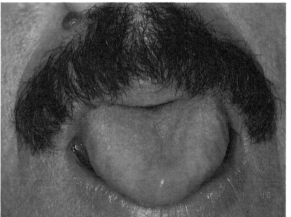

482 and 483 Hypothyroidism macroglossia before and after treatment. The large tongue seen in **482** may have aggravated the presenting symptom of snoring (which the patient, a TV sound engineer, had recorded!). Seven months later the tongue no longer touches the angles of the mouth and the indentations from the teeth are smaller (**483**). A big tongue may reflect a small mouth, Down's syndrome, acromegaly, amyloid, hypothyroidism, or tumour.

484

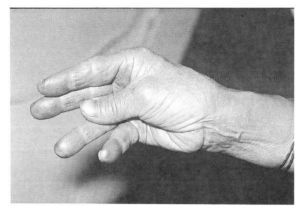

484 Carpal spasm (also known as 'accoucheur's hand' or Trousseau's sign*). The fingers are flexed at the mp joints, with the thumb adducted into the palm and the tips approximating. The brown pigment is henna, and the distended veins are the result of a sphygmomanometer cuff being applied on the arm to demonstrate the sign. Carpal spasm[18] is a manifestation of tetany; a contraction of distal muscles, usually in the hand (carpal) or foot (pedal spasm), though laryngeal spasm, too, may occur. The condition is a function of hyperexcitability of the peripheral nerve and may occur in hypocalcaemia,[19] hypomagnesiaemia, or with respiratory alkalosis, which leads to a fall in ionised calcium (hyperventilation). Idiopathic normocalcaemic tetany is termed spasmophilia.

485

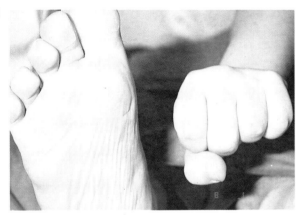

48

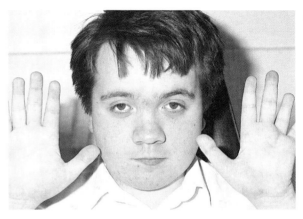

485 and 486 Pseudohypoparathyroidism—the sole of the foot with callus and the hand with a short metacarpal.[20] Callus is present over the 1st and 5th metatarsal heads, a reaction to local

weight transfer. The hands (**486**) have short 4th metacarpals and the face is characteristically broad and round. The stature is short.

487

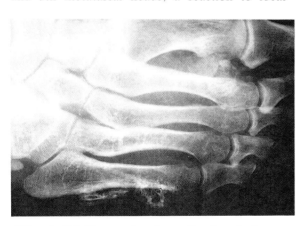

48

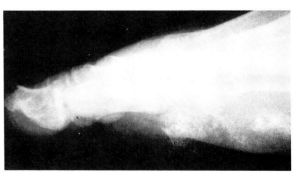

487 and 488 X-rays showing callus in relation to calcification. The callus overlays the aberrant soft tissue calcification—a feature of this hereditary condition manifesting the symptoms and signs of

hypoparathyroidism and associated with skeletal abnormalities. There is deficient end organ response to endogenous parathyroid hormone with consequent hyperplasia of the parathyroids.

*Armand Trousseau (1801–67), a French physician, described carpal spasm when a sphygmomanometer is pumped up above systolic pressure. He also gave his name to T's syndrome, with the spontaneous venous thrombosis of the upper and lower extremities in visceral cancer (see example in deep venous thrombosis section, **368**).

[18]Differential diagnosis of carpopedal spasm and tetany (**368**) fall in ionised calcium and the causes of hypocalcaemia—in this case, idiopathic hypoparathyroidism.

Adrenal

Excess adrenocortical hormones, endogenous or exogenous
- Excess cortisol—Cushing's* syndrome
- Excess aldosterone—aldosteronism
- Excess adrenal androgens—adrenal virilism.

Cushing's syndrome
A complex of fatigue, muscle weakness, amenorrhoea, hirsutes, purple striae, oedema, hypertension, glycosuria and osteoporosis. It may be ACTH-dependent—either from the pituitary or from another non-endocrine tumour—or ACTH-independent and related to adrenal hyper- or neo-plasia, or due to iatrogenic-manipulation. It is found predominantly (by a ratio of 3:1) in women. Clues in the leg may be sparse.

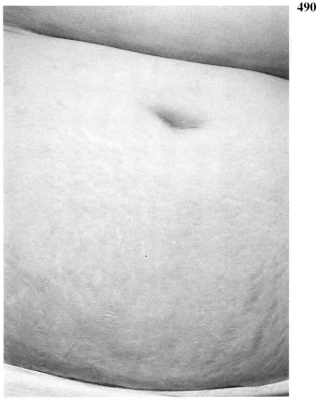

489 Livid striae on a leg. Skin striae present as narrow streaks or stripes of distinctive colour or texture (**489**). They are due to distraction of the skin structure due to lateral stretch, and may occur if the skin 'splits'—as when accommodating fat in weight gain, or in the case of the uterus in pregnancy, when they are coloured white and known as striae gravidarum (**490**). Abnormal fragility of skin collagen and thinning of the skin occur if there is an excess of corticosteroids, either applied as an ointment, secreted by the adrenal, or taken as medication, and livid striae and thinning of the skin may appear. The striae are seen over the legs, thighs, abdomen and buttocks. A common site is over the breasts in fat teenagers, when the striae may be livid initially—raising the question of Cushing's syndrome—before fading.

491 The skin of the ankle of an asthmatic on steroids, showing thinning and atrophy. There is an increased risk of damage.

[19]Hypocalcaemia—PTH ABSENT hereditary or acquired hypoparathyroidism, hypomagnesiaemia
—PTH INEFFECTIVE chronic renal failure, vitamin D lack or defective metabolism/diet or anticonvulsants, vit. D active/ineffective—malabsorption, end organ insensitive, pseudohypoparathyroidism
—PTH FLOODED acute hyperphosphataemia—tumour lysis, acute renal failure, rhabdomyolysis. Osteitis fibrosa after parathyroidectomy.
[20]Note that skeletal stigmata without biochemical abnormalities is termed pseudo pseudohypoparathyroidism!

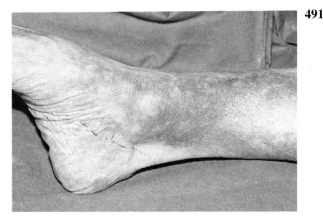

*Harvey Williams Cushing. American neurosurgeon, 1869–1939, described 1932.

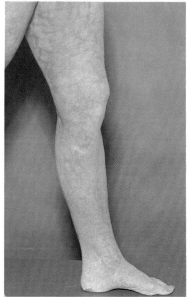

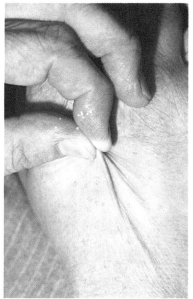

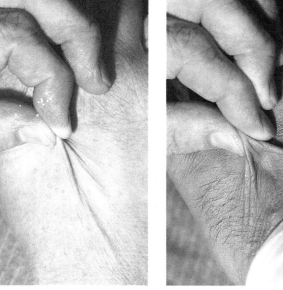

492 Livid striae on a leg.

493 and 494 Thin skin on the hand of a man with Cushing's syndrome (**493**) is compared with control skin (**494**).

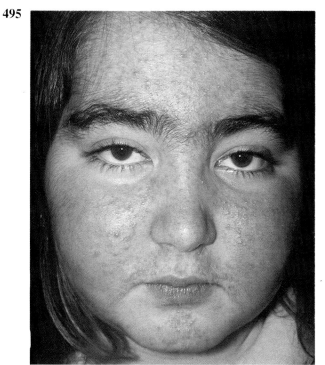

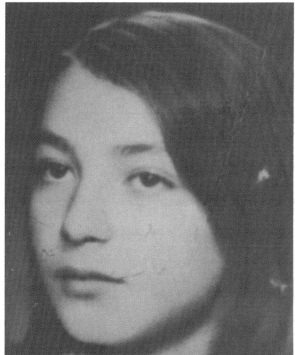

495–499 Cushing's facies. The girl in **495** is obese, plethoric, has acne and hirsutes, and is moon-faced. Note how she has changed from the picture taken a year earlier (**496**). In **497** and **498** the excess adrenal androgen leads to the need to shave; the hair is thinning and the face is rounded. The iatrogenic Cushing's seen in the 16-year-old boy in **499** developed during three months of steroid therapy: he is round-faced, with hirsutes, acne, thinning hair and facial plethora.

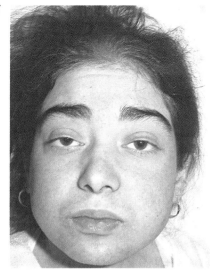
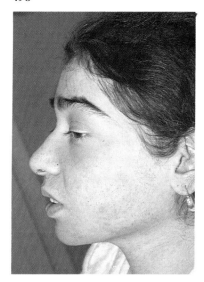
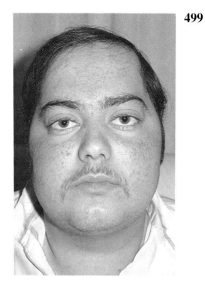

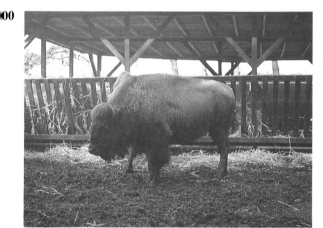
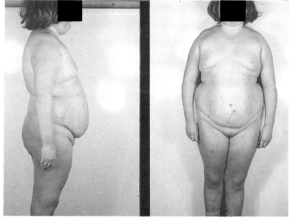

500 and 501 The buffalo with hump (**501**) shows the results of the deposition of fat over the upper torso, the truncal obesity leading to the creation of a 'buffalo hump'. The condition is associated with muscle wasting of the buttocks.

Adrenal insufficiency

A lack of cortisol leads to increased ACTH secretion and pigmentation.

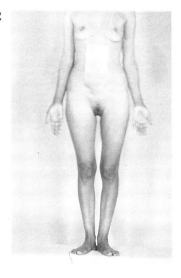

502

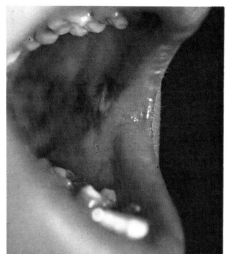

503

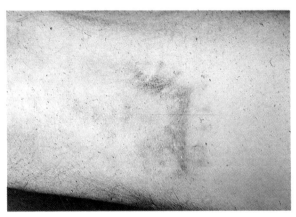

504

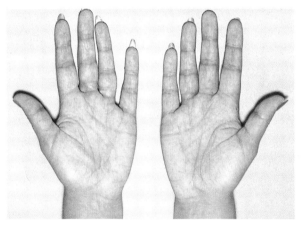

50

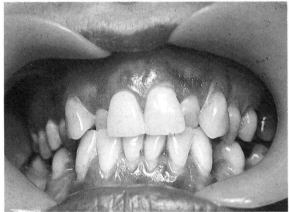

506

502 Full-length female pigmented legs. The pigmentation resembles sunburn (with which it may be mistaken). It is seen also in the mouth (**503 and 504**), in the palmar creases (**505**), and in scars which heal during the insidious onset of adrenal insufficiency (**506**). The pigmentation occurs often under the straps of underwear, but may be patchy (see **507**) and lead to a swarthiness of face. Vitiligo is present.

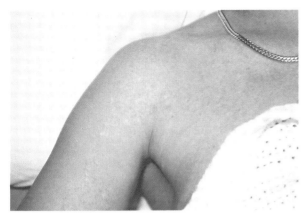

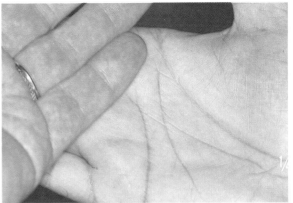

508

508–509 Pigmentation in the skin creases. Compare pigmentation due to ACTH excess (**505**) with that created racially (**508**) and by the application of a pigment such as henna (**509**).

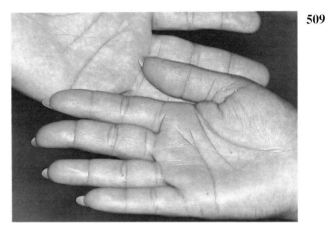

509

510 Vitiligo knee. Fifty per cent of patients with Addison's disease* have circulating adrenal antibodies, reflecting the auto-immune nature of the majority of cases—the remainder being due to granulomatous infiltration, tumour infiltration, sarcoid, amyloid or infarction. A marker of auto-immune disease may be the presence of vitiligo, which may be seen in association with adreno-cortical insufficiency, diabetes mellitus, hypothyroidism or pernicious anaemia.

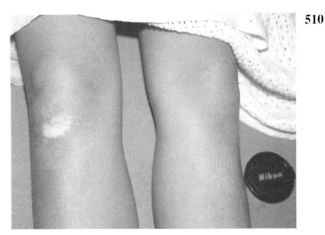

510

*After Sir Thomas Addison (1793–1860). Addison, T. 'Disease of the supra-renal capsules.' *London Hospital Gazette*, 1849, **43**: 517–8.

10 The foot in diabetes mellitus

Presentation Diverse—the manifestation of hyper-glycaemia or the result of one of its complications.

A *Local signs* which are suspicious
—of glycosuria
—of sepsis
—of local complications
         neuropathy—ulcers/joints
         ischaemia
         dry callus
         ulcers

B *Distant signs* which are confirmatory

C *Other presentations* which alert to the possibility of diabetes
—itching
—weight loss
—blurred vision
—skin signs of diabetes mellitus
—facies of other associated diseases:
         haemochromatosis
         Cushing's syndrome.

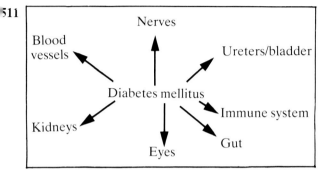

511 Systems affected.

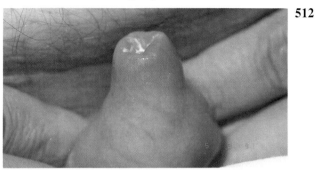

512 Phimosis and balanitis. Sugary urine leads to inflammation of the prepuce scarring to phimosis, often with *monilia*.

Local

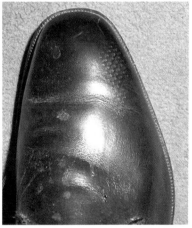

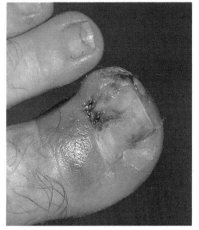

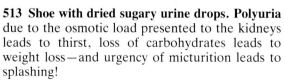

513 Shoe with dried sugary urine drops. Polyuria due to the osmotic load presented to the kidneys leads to thirst, loss of carbohydrates leads to weight loss—and urgency of micturition leads to splashing!

514 Typical acute onychocryphosis. The toe is infected and the nail folds are wide—exclude diabetes.

515 Chronic paronychia with inflammation of the surrounding nail, growth arrest line (Beau's line), and white areas where the nail has separated from the nail bed. Suspect diabetes.

516

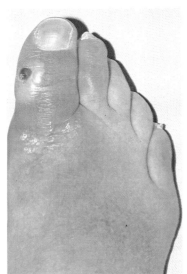

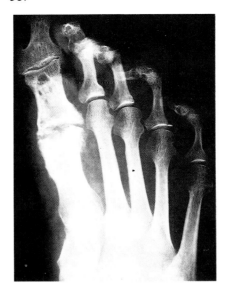

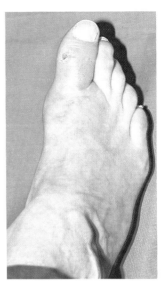

519

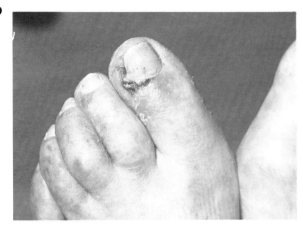

520

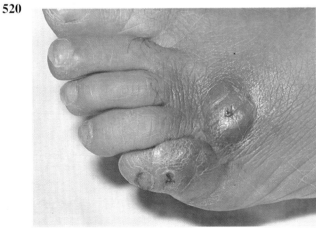

516 Infected toe in a diabetic man of 80 years. The dark area on the pocket of pus shows the site of the original abrasion over a fixed flexural deformity of the interphalangeal (IP) joints. Cellulitis has spread to the surrounding tissue.

517 An X-ray of the toe in **516** shows no bony involvement by the infection. Silastic implant at the 1st metatarsophalangeal (mtp) joint three years earlier.

518 The same foot as above, after healing.

519 A necrotic area at the base of a nail fold, in a diabetic with an ankle/brachial pressure index of 6·0[1], and rheumatoid arthritis. Mottling and oedema are present. This is **ischaemia** masquerading as sepsis. The patient died a few months later.

520 Infection on the dorsum of an atypical infected neuropathic foot: **chronic osteomyelitis** with a pressure lesion of the 5th toe.

[1] Ankle/brachial pressure index — normally.
$$\frac{\text{Systolic BP arm}}{\text{Systolic BP leg}} = 1.0$$

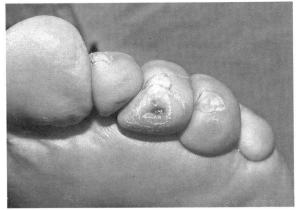

521 Flexural deformities of lesser toes, in a diabetic. There is bleeding into callus on the apex of the 3rd toe—a precursor to ulceration in **a neuropathic foot**.

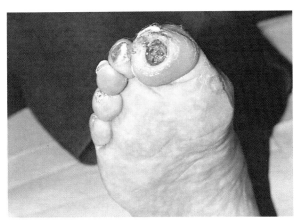

522 Fixed flexural deformity at the IP joint of the big toe, with ulceration following the initial blister. **Neuropathic foot**. Healed well.

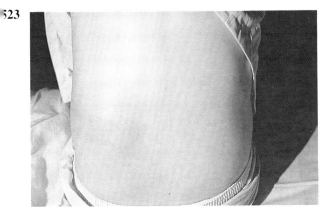

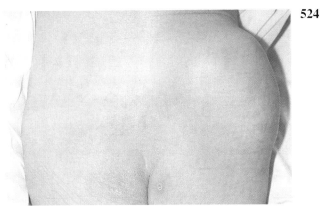

523 Abscess perinephric. Note the filling of the loin and the bulge with overlying redness. A diabetic presenting in pre-coma. Septic complications may be seen anywhere.

524 Abscess of the buttock. Weight loss and thirst culminated in presentation with sepsis. Note the small bedsore at the right edge of the natal cleft.

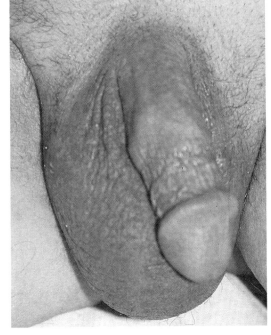

525 Recurrent pustules in a non-insulin dependent diabetic who squeezed lesions on the right groin and at each side of the scrotum. The underlying cause was eventually confirmed when the urine was tested for sugar.

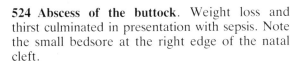

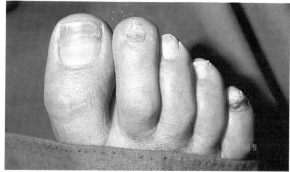

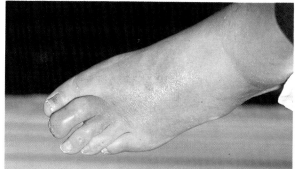

528

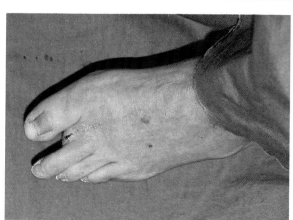

52

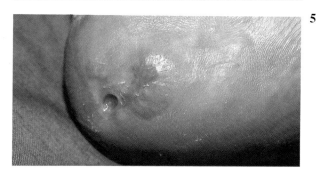

526 An ischaemic diabetic foot with a swollen 2nd toe and dystrophy of the nail. Exclude osteomyelitis in the distal phalanx. The growth arrest line on the big toe nail may reflect a period of ischaemia or local sepsis.

527 An infected ulcer on the apex of a swollen 2nd toe, with osteomyelitis and cellulitis extending on to the dorsum in **a neuropathic diabetic foot**.

528 The foot in **527** after **amputation of the 2nd toe**. The cellulitis has subsided and the incision healed.

529 An ischaemic diabetic foot with an indolent punched-out ulcer and sinus. Surrounding fibrous tissue scarring from previous ulceration—a typical site for ischaemic ulcers. No bony involvement at the lateral border of the foot.

530

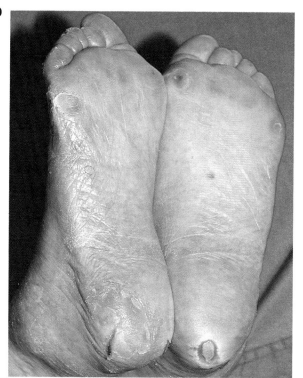

530 An ischaemic diabetic foot with thin shiny skin and a loss of fibro-fatty tissue over weight-bearing areas. Fissuring with little callus over both heels is a common site in ischaemic feet. On the heel one fissure has ulcerated.

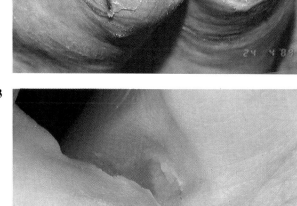

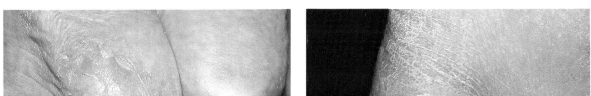

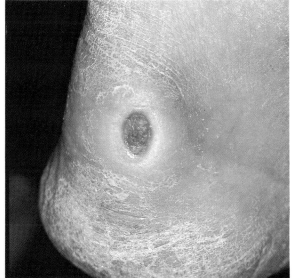

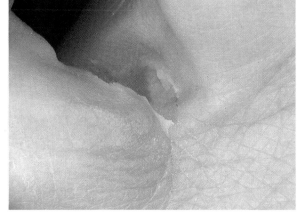

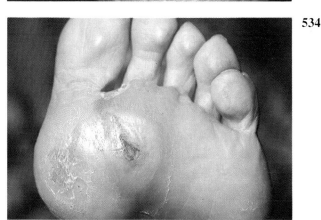

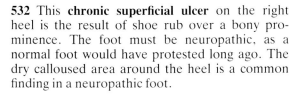

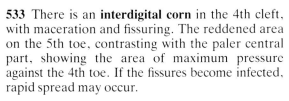

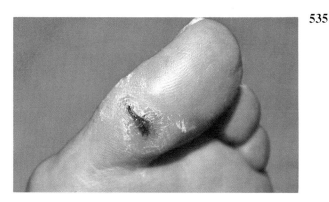

531 A close-up of the heels in **530**, showing **maceration around the ulcer** from exudate. Reddened areas on either side of the ulcer may also break down. Ankle oedema is present.

532 This **chronic superficial ulcer** on the right heel is the result of shoe rub over a bony prominence. The foot must be neuropathic, as a normal foot would have protested long ago. The dry calloused area around the heel is a common finding in a neuropathic foot.

533 There is an **interdigital corn** in the 4th cleft, with maceration and fissuring. The reddened area on the 5th toe, contrasting with the paler central part, showing the area of maximum pressure against the 4th toe. If the fissures become infected, rapid spread may occur.

534 A diabetic woman of 38 years, with **neuropathic feet**. Contours show a high weight load on the 1st and 2nd mt heads. She persistently wears court shoes. (Note moulding of pulps on 1, 2, 3, 4 toes.) Removal of callus over the 2nd mt head reveals an ulcer with superficial tracking to the 1st interdigital cleft, where scaling indicates the exit point for exudate.

535 Diabetic neuropathy with high weight loading over a fixed flexural deformity of the IP joints. Bleeding into callus frequently precedes ulceration.

536

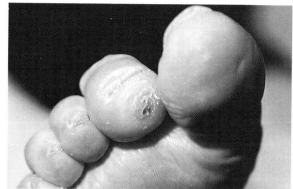

537

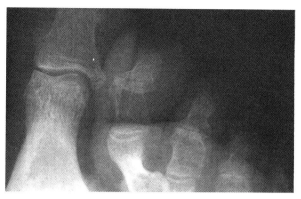

538

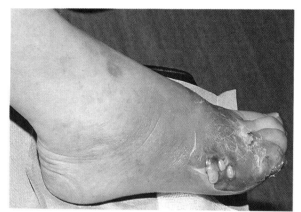

536 A swollen 2nd toe, with a sinus from **an ulcer discharging** through overlying callus in **a neuropathic diabetic foot**. Present for six months.

537 An X-ray of the toe in **536**, showing **osteomyelitis of the distal phalanx**.

538 A neuropathic diabetic foot. Infection from an interdigital fissure has spread on to the dorsum, with cellulitis and abscess formation. Complete resolution.

539

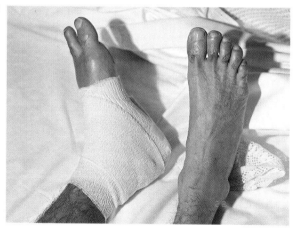

540

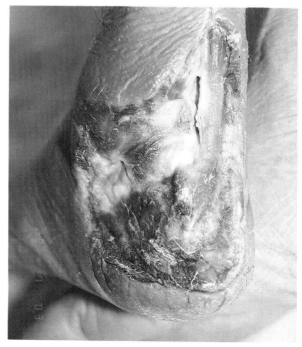

539 and 540 A Saudi aged 65 years. The innocuous appearance (**539**) hides a rapidly destructive anaerobic infection (**540**), which proves unresponsive to penicillin and is halted only by the appropriate treatment of anaerobic streptococci. A clue to the infection's presence is the characteristic musty smell.

541 and 542 A deep painless ulcer under the 2nd mtp is joint tracking to the 1st and 2nd interdigital clefts with cellulitis spreading to the dorsum. Infection has tracked into the 2nd toe via the flexor tendon sheath with osteomyelitis of the proximal phalanx. Persistent picking of the toe nails has caused nail dystrophy, not ischaemia — 'wilful self-neglect' nullifies routine medical care. The 2nd ray was amputated, but the patient did not return for the follow-up. There is a patch of necrobiosis lipoidica near the medial malleolus (**541**).

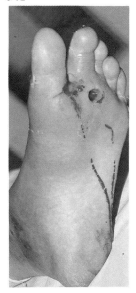
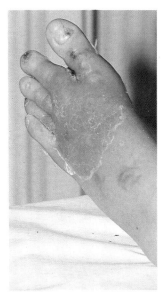

543 Diabetes was diagnosed three months earlier in this heavy smoker. Three weeks ago a fissure developed under the 1st toe, which became gangrenous and was amputated. The healing wound is illustrated.

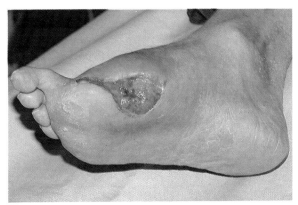

544 The same foot as in **543**, two months later, following kneeling while home decorating! There is **cellulitis** of the 2nd toe from apical ulceration, and **osteomyelitis of the distal and middle phalanges**. 2nd ray amputation was followed, later, by the 3rd and 4th rays.

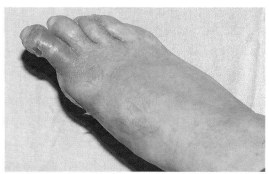

545

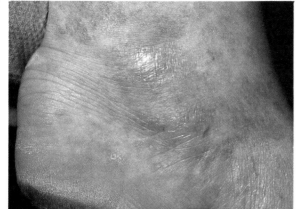

545–547 An obese diabetic woman with **ischaemic feet** (**545**) complained of pain in the heel when wearing shoes. An X-ray (**546**) showed no abnormality, but a bone scan (**547**) revealed a hot spot over the tender area, indicating inflammation. The condition settled.

546

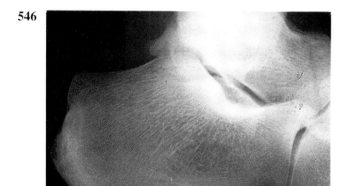

547

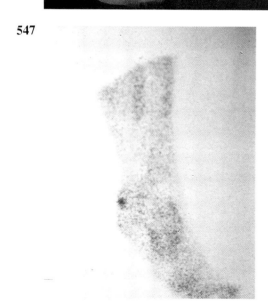

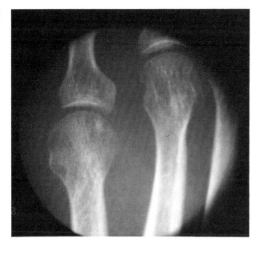

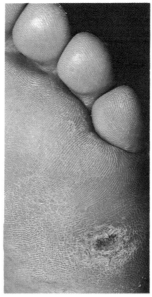

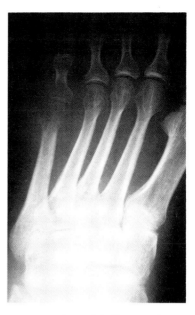

548–550 A non-insulin dependent diabetic man aged 60 complained of minor discomfort in the lateral foot. The X-ray (**548**) was normal. The foot was neuropathic with callus over the 5th mt head (**549**). There was no sign of inflammation. Discomfort persisted, however, and three weeks later another X-ray (**550**) confirmed osteomyelitis of the 5th mt head.

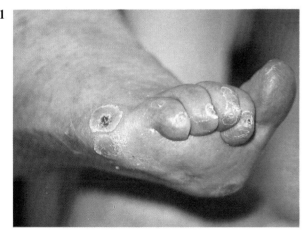

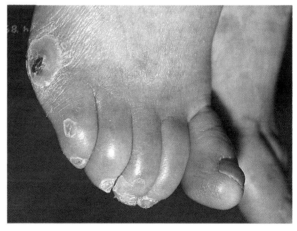

551–553 An ischaemic foot with a superficial ischaemic ulcer on a typical site—the lateral border near the 5th mt head (**551**). After lowering the foot the colour changes to the rubor of dependency and the toes appear swollen and shiny (**552**). There is callus over scar tissue near the 5th mt head (**553**). Ulceration will recur at sites of scarring.

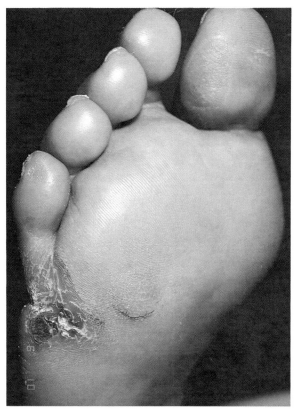

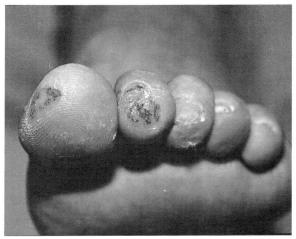

553 Wearing tight shoes has produced an oval area on the side of the big toe where it is pressed against the 2nd toe.

554 A neuropathic diabetic foot, with clawed toes and bleeding into the callus overlying the apices of the 1st and 2nd mt heads. A foot at risk.

555

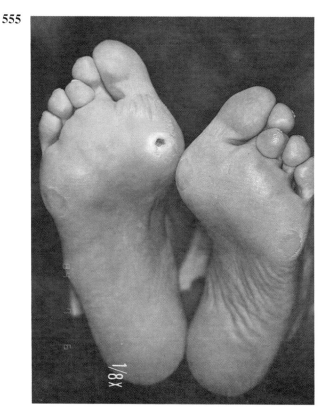

556

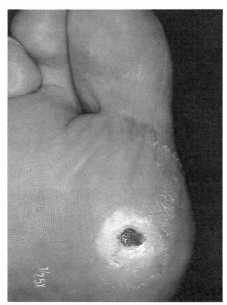

555 and 556 A highly arched diabetic foot with tight plantar fascia and a neuropathic ulcer on a common site—over the 1st mt head. A close-up (**556**) shows superficial ulceration.

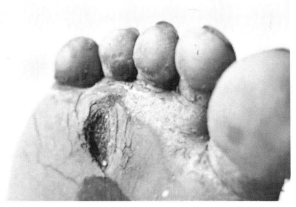

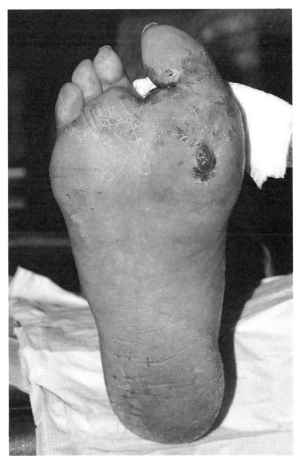

557 Tuberculoid leprosy: a perforating ulcer of the sole. Palpable nerves were felt in the neck and back of the hand.

A trophic ulcer related to sensory loss may also be seen in neuropathic conditions such as leprosy or tabes dorsalis, but here, by contrast, it is over the 3rd mt head (an uncommon site in a diabetic foot). Note that there is no toe retraction and that the foot is heavily calloused from walking bare foot.

558–560 An ulcer under the 1st mt head in a **diabetic neuropathic foot (558)**. The 2nd toe had been amputated and the 1st mt head was excised **(559)**—but the appearance of granulation tissue at the base of the ulcer and the application of silver nitrate suggested a complicating factor. The X-ray of the axial view **(560)** revealed **osteomyelitis in the sesamoid bones**.

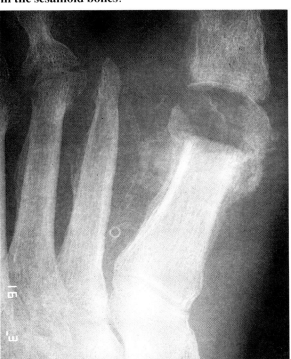

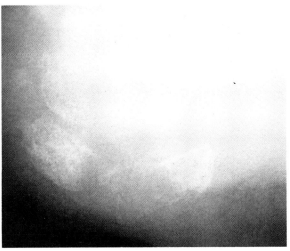

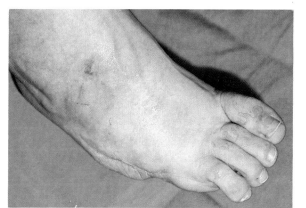

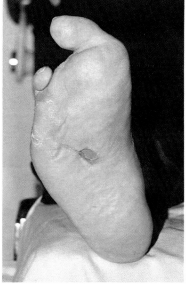

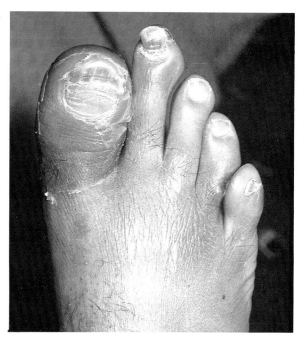

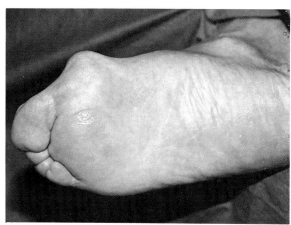

561 By contrast, a non-diabetic woman had poliomyelitis at the age of five, which resulted in a **plantar-flexed inverted forefoot** and painful over-loading of the 5th mt head. After excision of the 5th ray, a transfer lesion—a neuropathic ulcer—developed under the 4th mt head. Analgesic areas secondary to surgery exist on the lateral border and sweating ceases just proximal to the suture line. Neuropathic transfer lesion occurring in polio.

562 A diabetic neuropathic foot. A previous ulcer over the 5th mt head had tracked along the plantar fascia, forming an abscess on the sole of the foot. The 5th ray was removed because of osteomyelitis and a plantar incision made for drainage.

563 A diabetic on a drunken weekend in Rome fell asleep still wearing his new Italian shoes! The result was **exfoliation** around the swollen great toe and **discoloration** in the 4th cleft, with lateral compression of the long 2nd toe and its bulbous tip (reflecting the prolonged wearing of tight pointed-toe shoes). Note dystrophy of the 1st and 2nd nails (through a combination of shoe pressure and ischaemia).

564 A typical forefoot deformity in **hallus valgus**, with overloading of the 2nd mt head. If neuropathy develops in this diabetic foot, problems could result in this area of high loading.

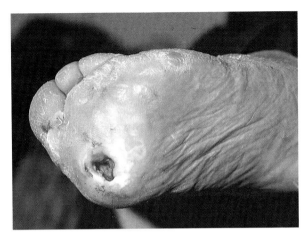

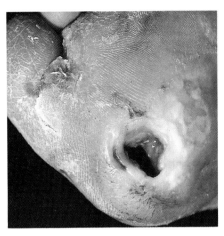

565 and 566 A neuropathic foot, with a chronic deep ulcer with surrounding macerated callus and fixed deformities of the toes (**565**). An X-ray showed no bony involvement with intact peri-osteum. A close-up view (**566**) shows the ulcer tracking medially. Peeling at the base of the great toe suggests shearing stress.

Ischaemic presentations

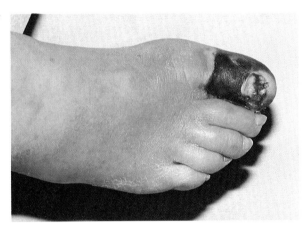

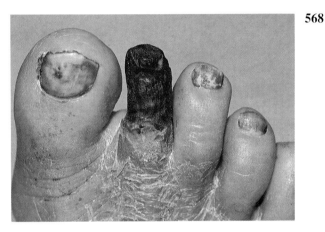

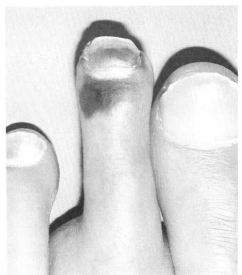

567 Diabetic moist gangrene of the big toe, related to infection with cellulitis and oedema of the surrounding tissues—as if the infection had outrun the blood supply and thrombosis of the vessels had led to gangrene.

568 Dry gangrene with mummification of the 2nd toe, in an ischaemic diabetic foot. No signs of infection; some scaling at the base of the 2nd toe prior to 'auto-amputation' (the toe falls off).

569 A long swollen 2nd toe with discoloration over the distal phalanx and under the nail. The ischaemic foot, with pre-gangrenous toes, mimicking bruising.

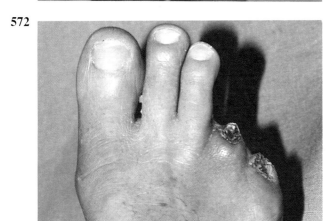

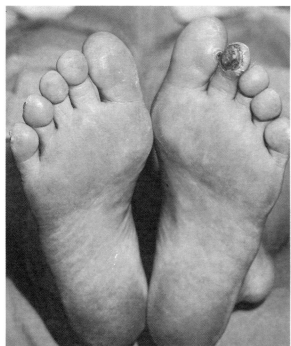

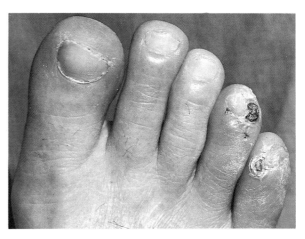

570–575 Diabetic ischaemic feet. The left foot is in peril with gangrene of the 2nd and 1st toes (**570**). There is patchy terminal gangrene of the 4th and 5th toes of the right foot (**571**).

Auto-amputation occurred nine months later on the right foot (**572**). On the other side, where the ischaemic toes and a gouty tophus can be seen in **573**, it followed ten months later (**574**). Note the circular white cross-section of calcified digital artery (arrow) and its calcification in the X-ray (**575**).

572

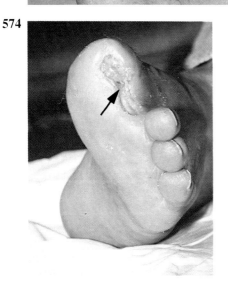

574

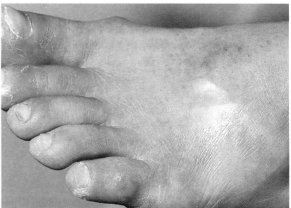

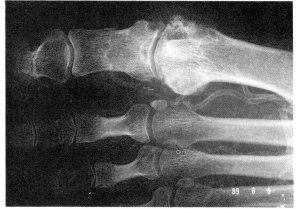

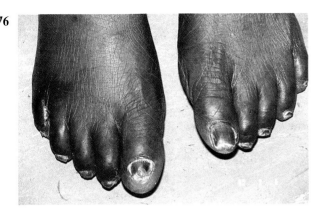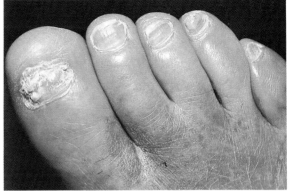

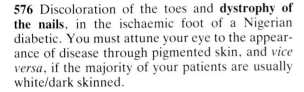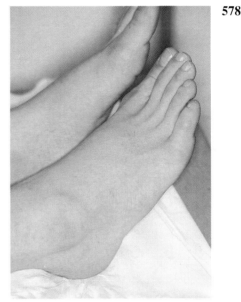

576 Discoloration of the toes and **dystrophy of the nails**, in the ischaemic foot of a Nigerian diabetic. You must attune your eye to the appearance of disease through pigmented skin, and *vice versa*, if the majority of your patients are usually white/dark skinned.

577 Dystrophic nails with growth arrest lines (Beau's* lines), in an ischaemic foot. Thin shiny hairless skin.

578 By contrast, the slim feet of a young male. Sweat from hyperhidrosis moistens the paper sheet. Sweaty feet are normal—no autonomic neuropathy and with less friction shear to produce callus. Increased sweating should stimulate questions as to the likely cause:

(i) Emotion/youth?
(ii) Fever/thyrotoxic/acromegalic?
(iii) Most pertinent: are the feet hypoglycaemic? (If your clinic is running late before lunch!)

579 The leg of a diabetic with neuropathy—pitting oedema being associated with autonomic neuropathy. **Diabetic autonomic neuropathy** with degeneration of the sympathetic nervous system may be manifest as:

- Postural hypertension
- Nocturnal diarrhoea
- Impotence
- Sweating after food
- Cardiac arrhythmia and cardiac arrest.

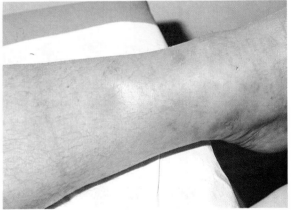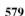

*Honoré Simion Beau, French physician, 1806–1865.

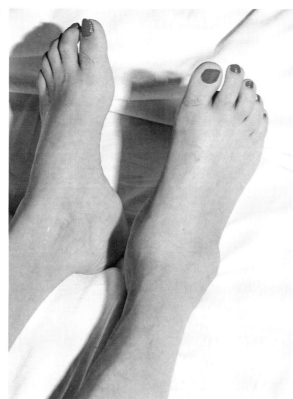

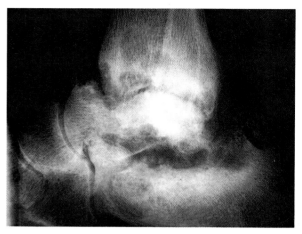

580 and 581 Neuropathic ankle joint. A diabetic with a left hemiplegia developed a right sub-talar neuropathic joint in her good limb, which had sustained a minor sprain at the kerbside, resulting in an osteoporotic trabecular fracture and starting the cycle of joint disorganisation seen in the X-ray (**581**).

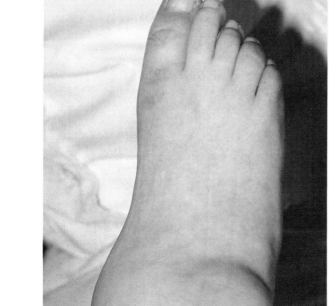

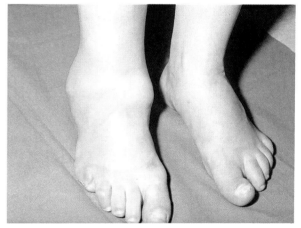

582 A very unstable **Charcot's ankle joint in a diabetic** woman aged 20 years, following a fracture of the lower end of the fibula three years earlier. A firm boot is necessary to stabilise the foot on walking. Excessive movement has caused nail problems on the lateral border of the big toe.

583 A Charcot's joint in a neuropathic diabetic. A warm foot with distended veins reflects arterio-venous shunting.

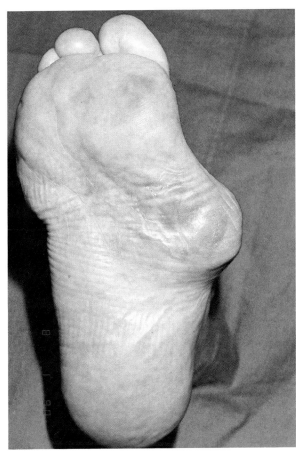

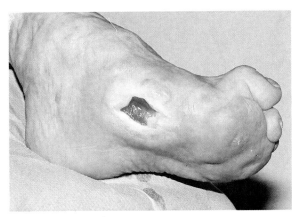

585

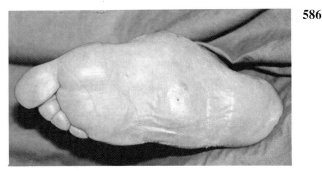

586

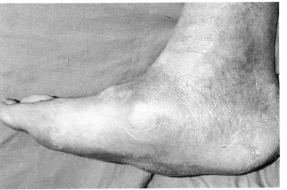

587

584 An insulin-dependent diabetic (one of the two brothers—see **586**), with a fixed neuropathic deformity which has never ulcerated or caused trouble.

585 A hypermobile Charcot's joint in the tarsal area of a neuropathic left foot. The foot is very mobile and pronates excessively, the medial ulcerated border taking the weight leading to a chronic superficial ulcer with an undermined edge and macerated callus from exudate. Autonomic neuropathy leads to a arterio-venous shunting with dilated veins at the ankle.

586 and 587 The brother of the insulin-dependent diabetic in **584** has **bilateral mid-tarsal rigid Charcot's joints** (**586**) and rocker bottom deformities (**587**) which periodically ulcerate over bony points.

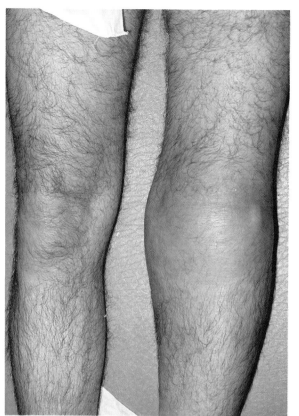

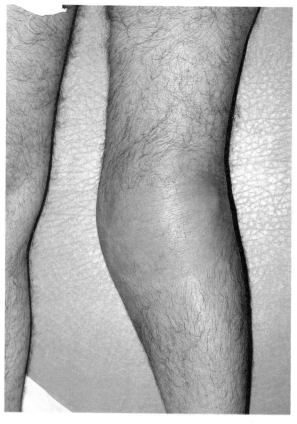

590

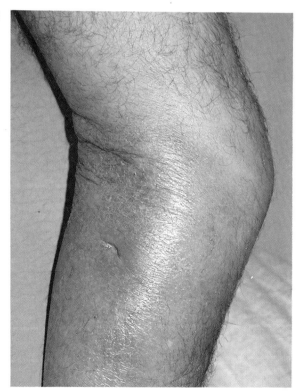

588–590 Tabes dorsalis—neurosyphilis. By contrast, the neuropathic joint[2] in the lower limb is usually the knee. There is secondary quadriceps-wasting here (**588**)—the knee is supported by a caliper. Although painless, it demonstrates an abnormal range of movement, which damages it further (**589**). Infection and sinus formation occurred three years later (**590**).

[2]Neuropathic joints occur when diminished pain sensation removes its protective cover in leprosy, syphilis and syringomyelia, with the additional complication of autonomic neuropathy and high vascular flow leading to porotic bone collapse in diabetes (described in 1868 by Jean Charcot [1825–93]. a French neurologist).

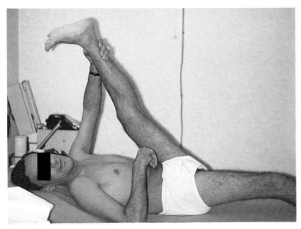

591

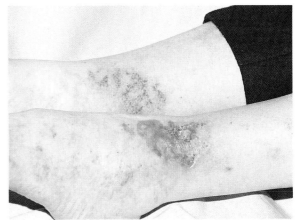

592

591 A man demonstrating that he has an abnormal range of movement. This could be normal—for example, if he were an acrobat or sat cross-legged all day with very mobile hips. It could be due to lax ligaments—Peter Pan hypermobility syndrome, for instance, or a disorder of collagen such as pseudoxanthoma elasticum. He could be hypotonic, due either to lower motor neuron paralysis, or to a cerebellar or posterior column lesion such as tabes dorsalis. He could have a disordered neuropathic joint with a painless abnormal range of movement.

He had bilateral ptosis—congenital, myopathic, tabetic or myaesthenic. Diagnosis: **tabes dorsalis**.

592 Diabetic neuropathy: painless burns from standing gossiping by a car exhaust!

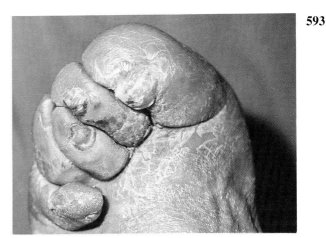

593

593 and 594 A diabetic foot with neuropathy. There are fixed deformities of all toes at the mtp and IP joints (**593**), making hygiene, and avoidance of interdigital maceration with fissuring, difficult. There is dry scaling skin with an absence of sweating, and also disordered keratinisation of the nails. The proximal base of the 2nd toe shows hyperkeratotic and verrucous changes found in lymph stasis (**594**). This prevents pinching up of a fold of skin over the dorsal aspect (Stemmer's sign).

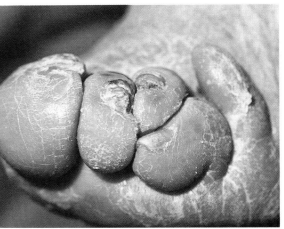

594

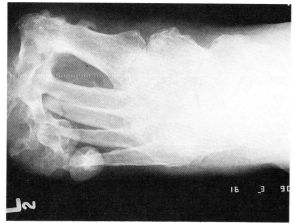

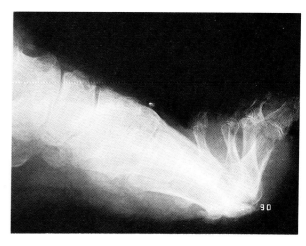

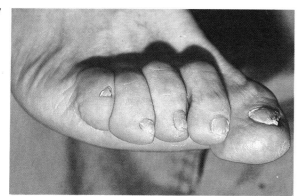

59

595 and 596 These two X-rays of the feet show classic changes in the diabetic foot with metatarsal attenuation and spindling associated with loss of differentiation between cortex and medulla and periosteal reaction.

597 Retracted toes due to weak intrinsic muscles (the 'intrinsic minus' foot) in diabetic neuropathy.

598 Diabetic amyotrophy. A recently diagnosed diabetic with pain and tenderness of the thighs associated with weakness and wasting—particularly of the anterior thigh muscles of the right leg. May be due to a femoral neuropathy, but its association with recent insulin use suggests a metabolic cause.

599 Meralgia paraesthetica. Also associated with pain, burning in quality, in the anterior thigh, this sensory neuropathy is related to compression of the lateral cutaneous nerve of the thigh (L 2, 3) beneath the inguinal ligament, and is frequently seen in diabetics. There is no muscle wasting. The area of abnormal sensation is mapped. May be associated with obesity or the wearing of a plaster corset, or sitting in bed after cardiac bypass surgery.

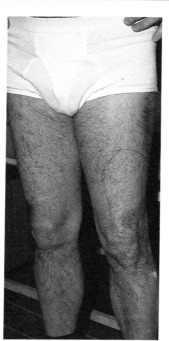

Complicationsof treatment

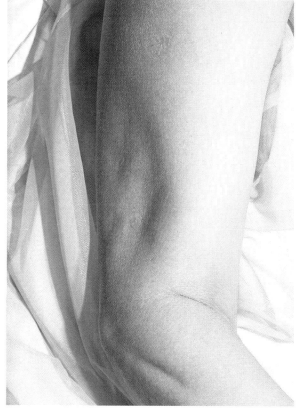

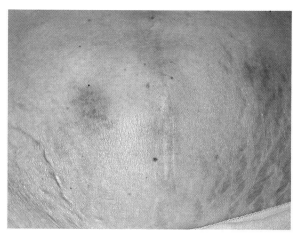

600 Insulin fat atrophy. At the site of repeat insulin injections, atrophy of the subcutaneous tissues produces a depression—although, occasionally, hypertrophy may occur. It is more frequently seen in (or complained of by) females. This woman, an insulin-dependent diabetic, spent three months in hospital with a stroke. The arm in question, being the one nearest to the door of her room, was that chosen by the nurse for injections.

601 Haemosiderin deposits, at the site of insulin injections on the abdomen in a cirrhotic diabetic with a prolonged prothrombin time.

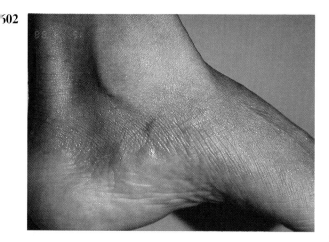

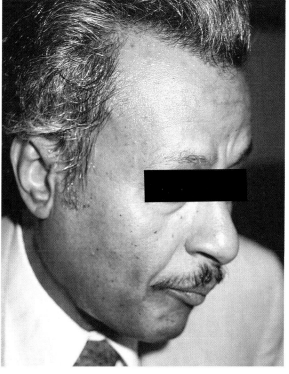

602 and 603 'Sweaty feet', as presented by an aggressive male diabetic who has missed his lunch. The sweat is clearly related to hypoglycaemia: see, think—and salvage with sugar! (Look at the forehead in **603**.)

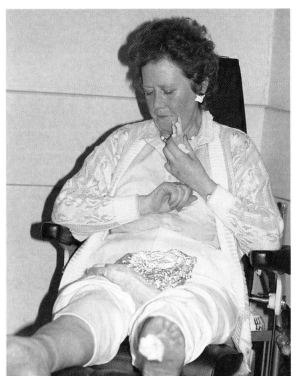

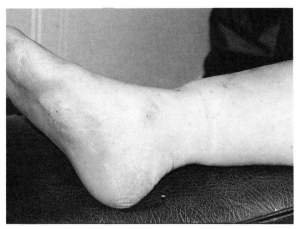

604 and 605 Hypoglycaemia. Midwinter, and a sweating diabetic who has missed a meal. The dew on the forehead due to sympathetic stimulation leads to tachycardia, sweating and dilated pupils. Treated with a snack (**604**), note how her sweating diminishes distally as her peripheral neuropathy increases (**605**). The moulding of the lower leg is due to boots worn to stabilise a mobile mid tarsal Charcot joint. The callus on the plantar aspect indicates site of loading.

Complications of the eye

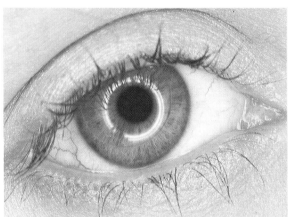

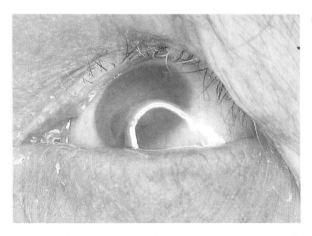

60

606 A normal eye with a contact lens. Bright cornea, matt pupil, no conjunctival infection— normal lashes.

607 Trachoma. Ground glass appearance of cornea overlying the pupil should not be confused with the milky white of an opaque cataract lens. Conjunctival scarring has led to ingrowing eyelashes which aggravate the corneal problem.

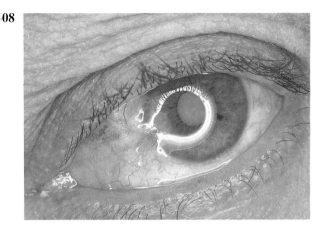

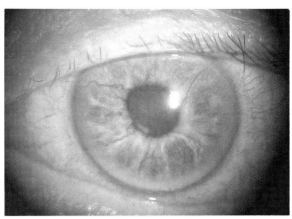

608 Cataracts occur earlier in diabetics than in members of the general population. Other causes of cataracts include trauma, ionising radiation, dystrophia myotonica, hypocalcaemia, and steroid therapy.

609 Rubeotic iris. New vessel formation over the iris must mean neovascularisation in response to ischaemia, whose cause may be diabetes, arteritis, carotid artery disease or any condition leading to ocular ischaemia. There are new vessels and ciliary injection, corneal oedema (dull) and a corneal arcus present—a picture of glaucoma.

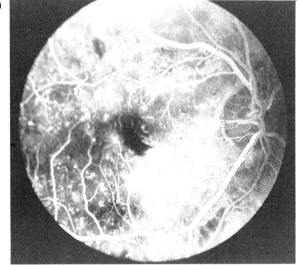

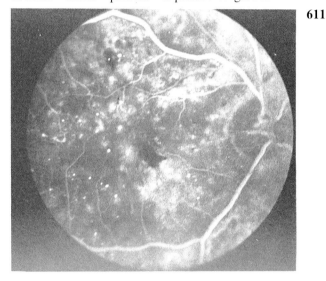

610 and 611 Angiograms of the fundus, showing leakage of dye (**610**) and micro-aneurysms (**611**) in a diabetic.

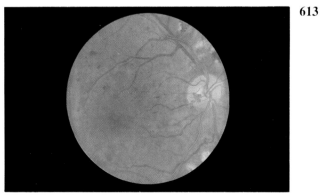

612 Early background diabetic retinopathy, with microaneurysms and haemorrhages.

613 Diabetic retinopathy, with haemorrhages, microaneurysms and new vessel formation (neovascularisation) on the disc.

614

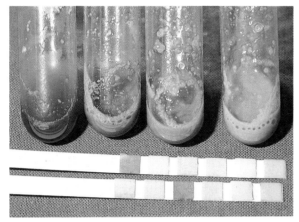

614 Glycosuria. The test tubes contain, from left to right, respectively, 0%, ½%, 1% and 2% glucose in urine. The colour change occurs when urine is added to Benedict's reagent or a Clinitest tablet: if a reducing substance is present, the copper sulphate in the solution is converted to cuprous oxide on heating, causing the colour to change, through green (½%) to orange (2%).

Dipstick tests with paper impregnated by reagents are convenient. Normal stix above, and dipped in glucose containing urine below. Other filter squares indicate (left to right) pH and the presence of albumen, sugar, ketones, blood.

Cutaneous associations

The presence of these cutaneous changes should prompt the testing of the urine for sugar.

615

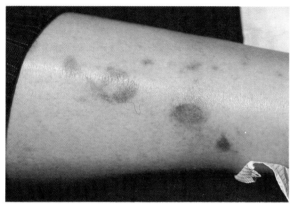

615 Diabetic dermopathy begins as a dull red papule on the front of the leg; the papule may blister. It progresses to a dried central scale (see

61

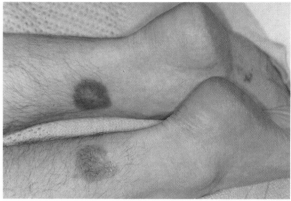

centre of picture), which leaves a depressed scar (left of picture). The pigment is haemosiderin. It may be associated with microangiopathy.

617

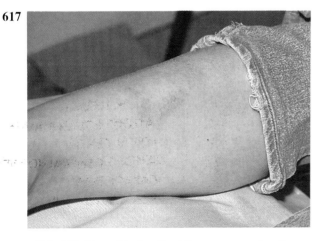

61

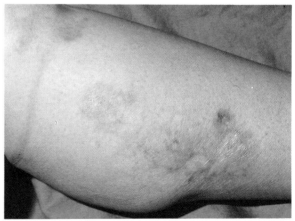

616–618 Necrobiosis lipoidica occurs in three diabetics in a thousand but is not confined to this group. The oval indurated plaque, with a depressed atrophic centre varying in colour, may ulcerate, and can co-exist with granuloma annulare. The constriction line seen in **619** is due to a garter.

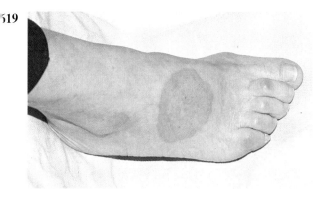

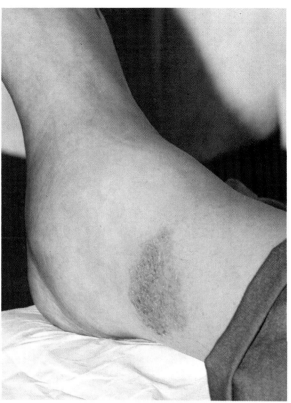

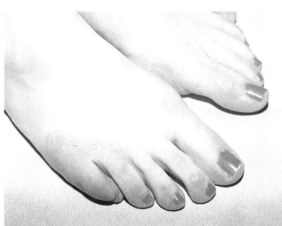

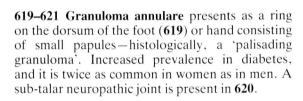

622

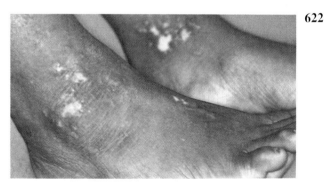

619–621 Granuloma annulare presents as a ring on the dorsum of the foot (**619**) or hand consisting of small papules—histologically, a 'palisading granuloma'. Increased prevalence in diabetes, and it is twice as common in women as in men. A sub-talar neuropathic joint is present in **620**.

622 Lichen planus presents with violaceous shiny feet topped with papules. It is usually seen at the ankle, but the wrist, mouth, penis, nail or hair may be affected. Increased incidence of abnormal glucose tolerance.

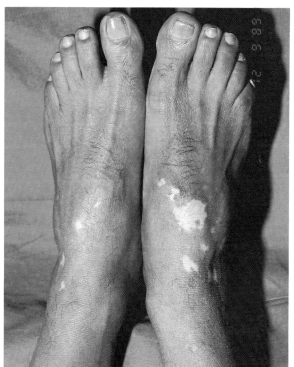

62

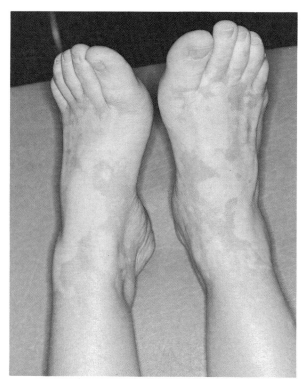

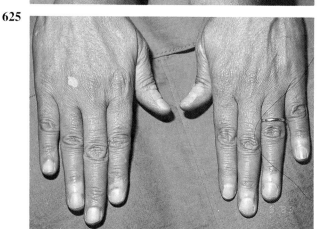

623–625 Vitiligo. Depigmentation of the skin, often symmetrical, is seen on the feet (**623 and 624**), legs, hands (**625**) or face, in association with other auto-immune conditions—diabetes, hypo/hyper thyroidism, Addison's disease and pernicious anaemia. The appearance on a pigmented skin may be very distressing to the patient. Compare with leprosy, where the depigmentation is incomplete.

626

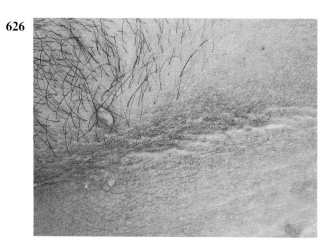

626 Acanthosis nigricans. Presents as velvety thickened flat pigmented areas, with skin tags, often in flexures of the neck, groin, axillae or soles of the feet. It is seen in obesity, in association with diabetes, and as a skin marker of an underlying adrenocarcinoma in the elderly.

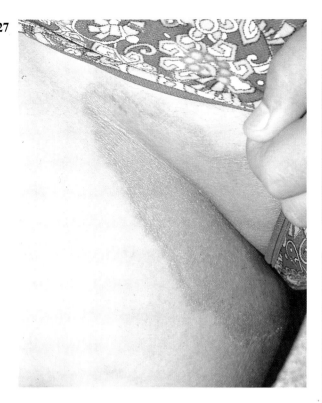

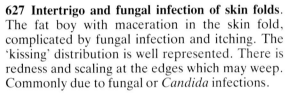

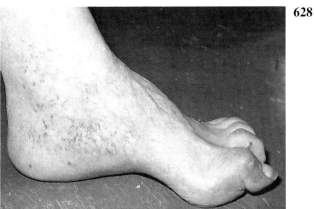

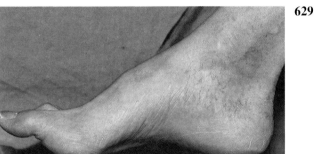

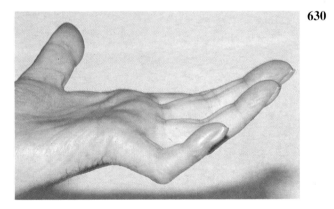

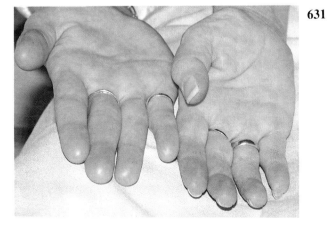

627 Intertrigo and fungal infection of skin folds. The fat boy with maceration in the skin fold, complicated by fungal infection and itching. The 'kissing' distribution is well represented. There is redness and scaling at the edges which may weep. Commonly due to fungal or *Candida* infections.

628 and 629 Glycosylation of collagen. This leads to tight plantar fascia and weak intrinsic muscles, which in turn lead to clawing of the toes. The 'intrinsic minus' foot. A neuropathic foot.

630 and 631 Diabetic cheiropathy. Tight stiff hands reflect the foot (see **629**). The subject's inability to extend the palm fully (**630**) contrasts with her normal unmarried daughter, whose hands are supple and moist (**631**). The hand is dry and the thenar eminence, particularly abductor pollicis brevis, is wasted due to neuropathy. Trigger finger is common in diabetes.

632

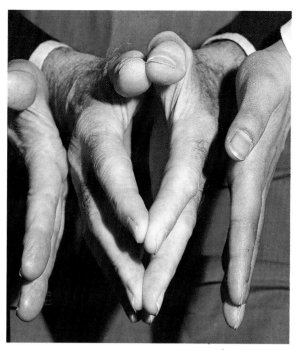

632 Cheiropathy and neuropathic feet. A Greek with IDDM is attempting to approximate the palms (see centre pair of hands in picture) but cannot in spite of exerting considerable force—note the index tips. Compare with the hand of a 22-year-old girl on his left and that of a 60-year-old woman on his right.

633

63

635

63

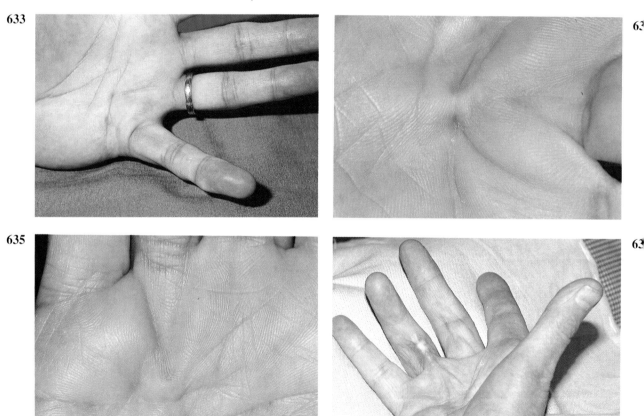

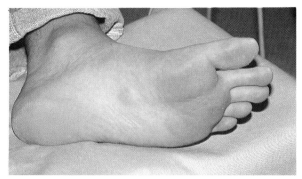

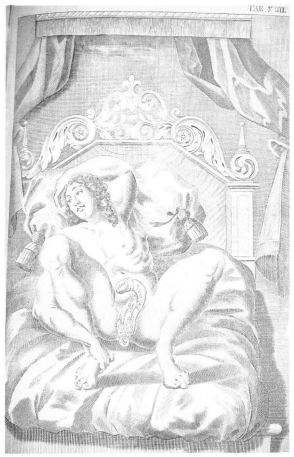

TAB. XIII. **638**

633–638 Dupuytren's contracture. Contracture of the palmar fascia as an initial tethering at one end of spectrum (**633**) to tying down of the finger in the palm at the other (**636**). The condition is associated with fibrotic conditions elsewhere — plantar nodules in the fascia of the sole (**637**) give little trouble and may be overlooked, unless pointed out by the patient who, in **638**, also demonstrates penile chordee with fibrous plaques in the corpora cavernosa, and angulation on penile erection.[3] Dupuytren's contracture is associated with alcohol abuse, trauma and anti-convulsant therapy; its incidence increases with age.

Renal complications

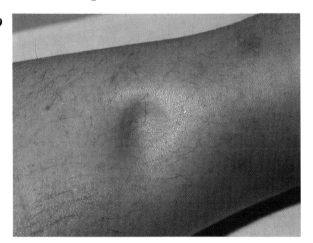

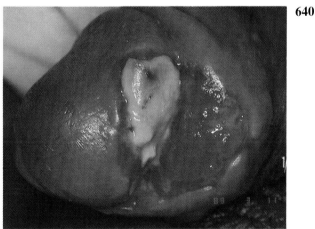

639 Oedema of the leg in a diabetic. Diabetic mellitus may be associated with increased incidence of urine infection, renal papillary necrosis, glomerular disease with proteinuria leading to hypertension and renal failure, or the nephrotic syndrome and oedema. Occasionally, oedema is seen in association with an autonomic neuropathy.

640 Ischaemic changes may produce ulceration and tissue destruction in **the diabetic penis** or balanitis (**512**).

[3]*Brown's Anatomy*, 1705 (2nd edn.).

641

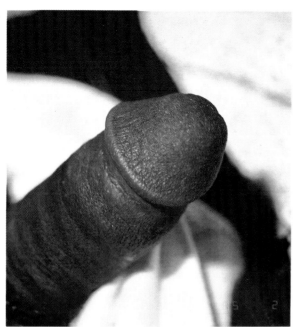

641 A penis with prosthesis inserted: **diabetic autonomic neuropathy** may lead to impotence. It is important to appreciate that many apparently inexplicable complaints may in fact have anxiety about impotence as their basis. Psychogenic causes must be excluded. Other manifestations of diabetic autonomic neuropathy are:

- Postural hypotension
- Nocturnal diarrhoea
- Gustatory sweating
- Hypoglycaemic unawareness
- Syncope associated with cardiac arrhythmias
- Decreased sweating of the feet.

642

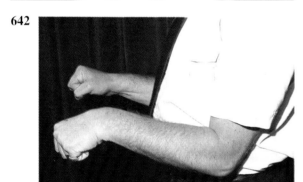

642–646 Mononeuropathies. Diabetic nerves are vulnerable. An isolated peripheral nerve palsy due either to mechanical compression over the arm of a chair (radial nerve palsy—**642**), which may lead to wrist drop, with an inability to extend the wrist joint on making a fist, or to pressure at the head of the fibula (**643**), leading to foot drop, with an inability to evert and dorsiflex the ankle.

643

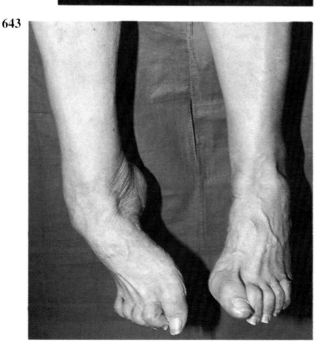

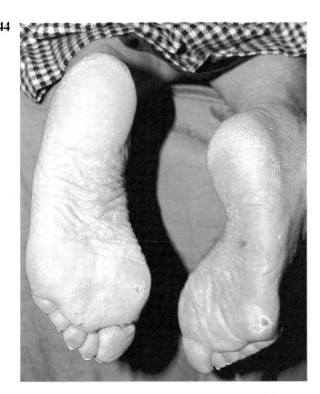

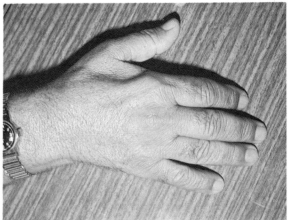

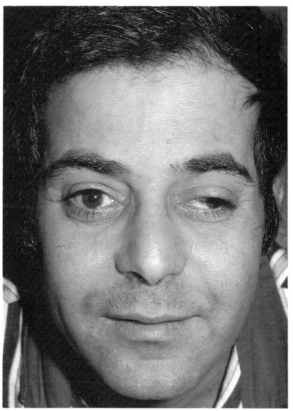

In the latter case, weight is taken over the 5th mt head (**644**).

Wasting of the interossei (**645**) may be due to a motor peripheral neuropathy in an isolated ulnar nerve lesion—note the guttering where the 1st dorsal interosseous should be. The subject here was a diabetic who had a left hemiplegia. His nurse had thoughtfully moved his watch to his right hand so he could refer to it—but placed it so that only she could read it with ease!

A median nerve lesion must not be assumed to be due to diabetes. Carpal tunnel compression of the nerve may occur and respond to decompression. A 3rd cranial nerve palsy may result in a squint, with the eye deviated laterally and downwards (**646**). This may be seen in middle-aged diabetics, but other causes must be excluded (they are best approached anatomically as the nerve has such a long intracranial course).

Nuclear:	—demyelinating disease
Midbrain:	—vascular infarct
Interpeduncular:	—arterial aneurysm
Cavernous sinus:	—fistula
Orbit:	—tumour, etc

No More Ignorance Coming Out.

647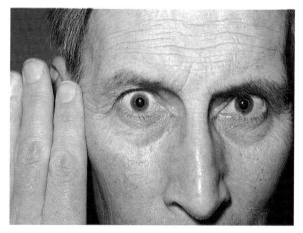

647 Haemochromatosis: bronze diabetic. Haemochromatosis is probably a genetic disorder— note the slate grey skin of the face compared with that of the control hand—associated with cirrhosis, diabetes and hypergonadism. May affect the joints and, in particular, the feet.

Glycosuria may be due to hyperglycaemia or renal glycosuria with a leak at normal blood sugar levels.

Lagstorage may result in a peak of hyperglycaemia exceeding the transport maxima in the kidney for glucose, and may also produce glycosuria. Proven diabetes mellitus must not prevent the clinician looking for a second basic pathology, such as, for haemochromatosis, bronze diabetes or Cushing's syndrome (steroid excess).

Finally: discovering diabetic mellitus and glycosuria must not blind you to a primary pathology.

11 The foot and circulation

Recognition of the foot 'at risk' from an impaired circulation

What physical signs are a pointer to an upset in the circulation of the feet? Look for changes in:

- Colour
- Texture
- Temperature
- Atrophy of skin
- Dystrophy of nails
- Atrophy of skin appendages
- Size
- Arterial pulse.

Impaired arterial circulation

648 Pallor of the foot. A child with acute leukaemia (Hb 5.0g%), next to a normal hand for comparison. Pallor depends on skin pigmentation, and on the thickness—as this determines the visibility of the capillary bed—as well as on the concentration of haemoglobin. In the hand, the nail bed is a useful colour chart for comparison with the examiner's hand (whereas, in the foot, the toe nail may be thickened or discoloured).

649 Unilateral growth arrest line and henna stain, seen in a man with auricular fibrillation, who had a popliteal artery embolism from left atrial thrombus. Brown stain on the nails is henna applied to toughen the skin (he is an Arabian gulf seaman). The nail growth which has occurred since his embolism is less on the left foot than on the right (by a ratio of 1.0:1.2), which can be judged from the henna stain. The slowing down in nail growth is due to the ischaemia, and to the appearance of a growth arrest line (Beau's lines*) on the toe nails of the affected foot. The time that has passed since the event can be estimated from the nail growth of about 5mm (0.5mm a week) that has occurred since the event—toe nails grow at about half to a third of the rate of finger nails. Ischaemia may lead to hair loss, too, but in this case the skin would have a shiny atrophic appearance (as in **650**). The hair 'loss' here is not a sign of value, being unconfirmed by any other change; in fact, the hairless appearance was simply due to shaving prior to arteriography!

Search for signs which may give a clue to the anatomical lesion, and then for a cause or predisposing factor for that anatomical lesion.

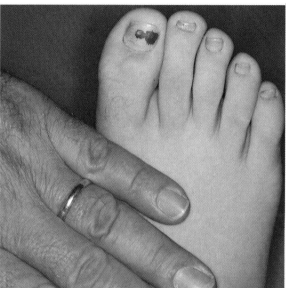

648

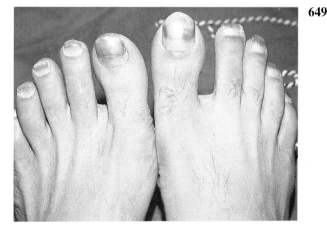

649

*Honoré Simon Beau (1806–65) described growth arrest lines in 1846. They are due to the slowing of nail growth which may occur with a systemic illness, an infectious fever such as measles or local ischaemia.

650

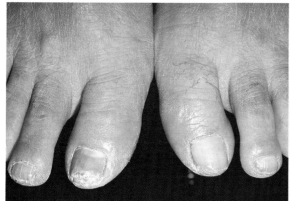

652

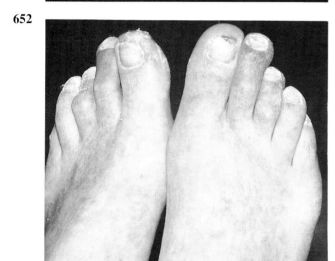

653

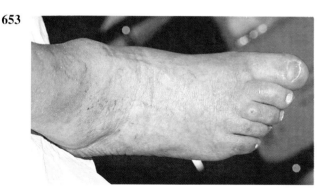

654

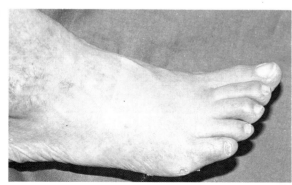

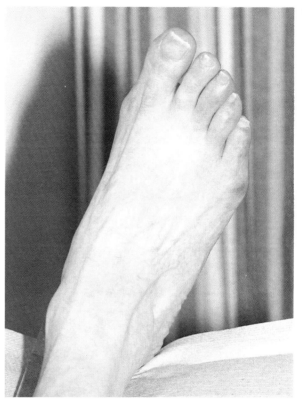

650 Thromboangiitis obliterans (Buerger's disease*). Early ischaemia of the feet with changes in the skin, which is shiny, dry, and a red colour—when dependent. The sweat glands atrophy and hair is sparse—particularly on the right foot, where there are nail changes and pulp atrophy of the great toe.

651 An ischaemic colour change of toes and a pressure lesion over the 5th metatarsal (mt) head, a common site (see **654**).

652 Ischaemic toes, nail changes and mottled skin. A stage on from **650**. The nails are thick and slow-growing, the skin dry and blanching with pressure —but the capillaries refill slowly.

653 Ischaemic toes on an elderly foot, with nail changes in the 5th toe.

654 An ischaemic foot. The lateral side of the 5th mt head has ulcerated—compare with **653**. The nails are dystrophic.

*Buerger, Leo (1879–1943). 'Thrombo-angiitis obliterans: a study of the vascular lesions leading to presenile spontaneous gangrene.' *Am. J. Med. Sc.*, 1908, **136**: 567–80.

184

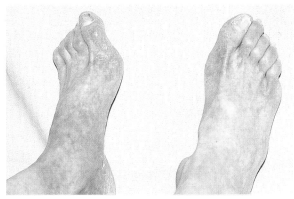

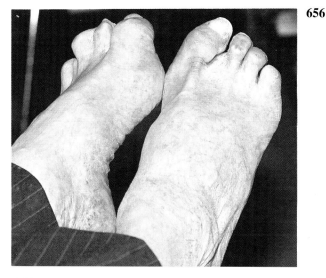

655 Mottled skin and retracted toes. Atrophy of the subcutaneous tissue leads to loss of fibro-fatty padding and the retraction concentrates weight over unprotected bony prominences.

656 Loss of the right 2nd toe. The toes are clawed at the interphalangeal (IP) joints and retracted at the metatarsophalangeal (mtp) joint. There is pulp atrophy and soft tissue loss.

657 and 658 Dorsal and plantar aspects of an ischaemic foot. The skin is thin and shiny. Fungus infection is present in the great toe nail and the tip of the 3rd toe has been lost (**657**). A pressure lesion is present over the lateral 5th toe. On the sole (**658**), the 2nd toe is clawed and has callus on the apex. There is a loss of plantar padding, and callus has formed over the 5th mt head, with underlying bleeding.

659 Thromboangiitis obliterans, presenting with nail dystrophy, dry skin, and the loss of the great toe of the left foot. This inflammatory disease of small/medium-sized arteries and veins affects the distal part of the arms and legs, leading to segmental occlusion. It occurs in men aged 20–40 years, frequently of Asian or Eastern European origin—there is an increased incidence of HLA-A9 and HLA-B5 antigens and cigarette smoking. There is peripheral ischaemia with claudication. Raynaud's phenomenon and superficial thrombophlebitis may occur. Digital ischaemia leads to pulp loss, nail changes, and gangrene.

657

658

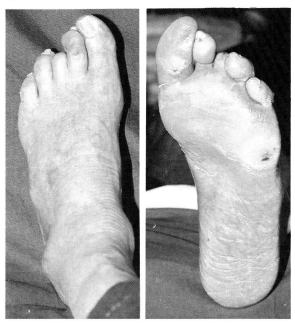

659

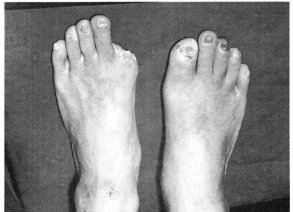

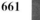

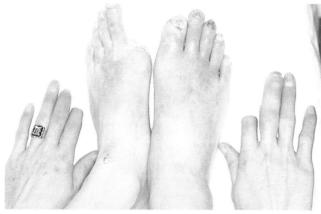

660 Thromboangiitis obliterans in a young Chinese cook. A heavy cigarette smoker with nail dystrophy, loss of fingers and toes, and nicotine staining at the level of loss: all clearly indicate poor patient compliance with the physician's advice! He drives a taxi with stick shift gearbox. How can you tell? See **602**.

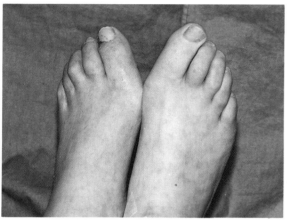

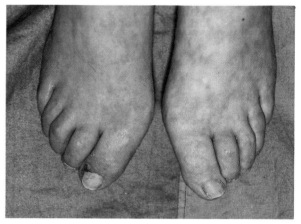

661 and 662 Severe vascular insufficiency: the effect of elevation and dependency. The foot blanches when it is raised above the level of the heart (**661**), and becomes mottled when lowered below that level (**662**). There is an ischaemic area at the base of the left great toe.

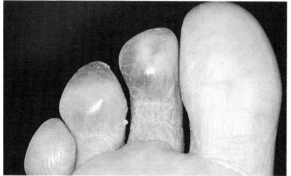

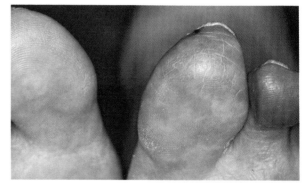

663 and 664 Severe vascular insufficiency. The mottled toe tips blanch on pressure (**663**) but show delay of capillary refilling once that pressure is released. Compare with chilblains (**664**).

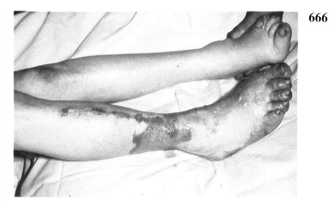

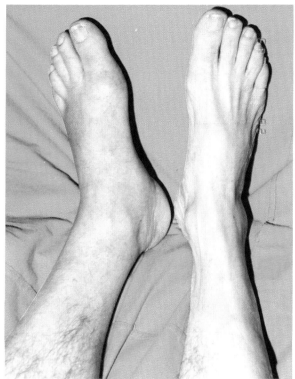

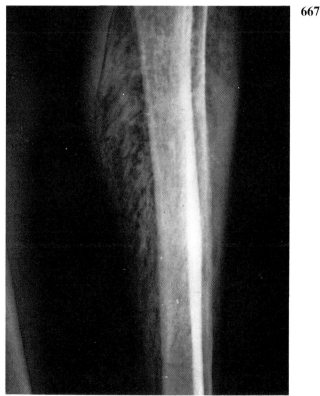

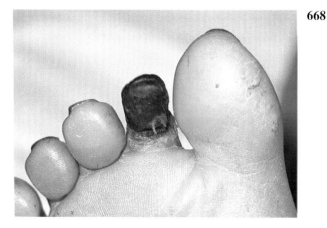

665 Venous mottling and swelling due to venous engorgement from a left deep vein thrombosis.

666 Acute arterial obstruction. There is an arterial embolus of the right leg; gangrene is incipient. Presents with sudden pain, paralysis, paraesthesiae, pulselessness and pallor.

667 An X-ray of the lower leg, showing the presence of gas between the planes of the muscles of the calf and outlining the tissues. This man had atrial fibrillation and sustained a saddle embolus. The legs were excoriated and a mixture of herb and cow dung was applied by a herbalist. Gas gangrene ensued in the dead tissue.

668 Auto-amputation of the 2nd toe. This ischaemic toe has developed a line of separation and will dry and fall off.

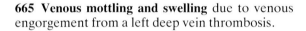

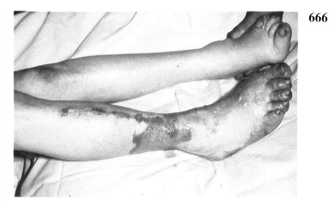
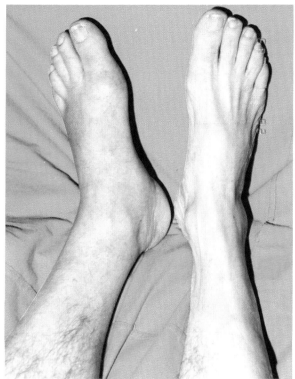
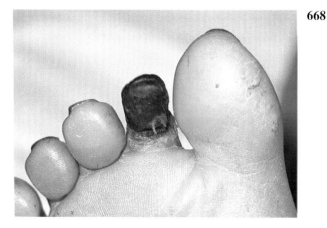

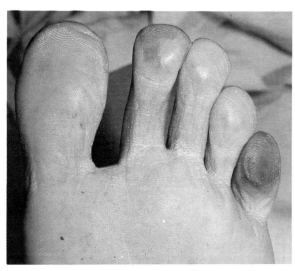

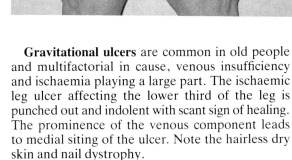

669 and 670 Gangrene of the pulp of the 5th toe (669) and the finger tips (670). Cutaneous ischaemic changes may reflect systemic disease. In systemic lupus erythematosus, digitial gangrene due to small vessel infarct may occur or develop with severe Raynaud's phenomenon.

Gravitational ulcers are common in old people and multifactorial in cause, venous insufficiency and ischaemia playing a large part. The ischaemic leg ulcer affecting the lower third of the leg is punched out and indolent with scant sign of healing. The prominence of the venous component leads to medial siting of the ulcer. Note the hairless dry skin and nail dystrophy.

671–674 Gravitational leg ulcers. These patients all attend 'an ulcer clinic in a slum backstreet'; they are predominantly female and often multi-parous, elderly, obese, immobile, and poor. These social factors are all crucial to their problem.

671

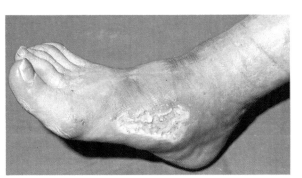

671 Ulcer medial ankle. An immobile foot. Fibrosis and scarring are seen proximal to the punched-out indolent ulcer, which may have begun over minor trauma over the tibia. Subcutaneous fibrosis is present in the upper leg.

672

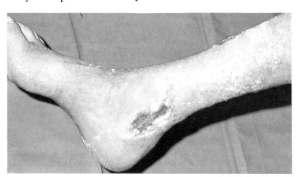

672 Ulcer medial foot, of an elderly pensioner who sits in her room all day. There is oedema due to recurrent inflammation and fibrosis in the subcutaneous tissues, with verrucous changes over the instep. The toes are shiny and mottled with a patch of atrophie blanche* at the base of the 2nd and 3rd toes. The foot has rolled into valgus, and shoe pressure broke the skin—leading to ulceration. Healing is now occurring. The discoloration is accentuated by applied pastes.

*Obliteration of capillaries in the upper dermis causing sclerosis. The residual vessels are attenuated and liable to thrombosis and consequent ulceration.

673 Ulcer medial malleolus. The pulses were not felt and the appearance is ischaemic.

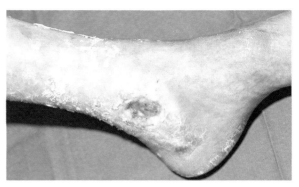

673

674 Ulcer lateral malleolus. The feet are neglected, with uncut toe-nails. A lateral site is less common, more usually ischaemic, and often associated with minor trauma.

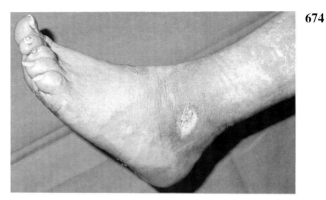

674

Markers of risk

Hyperlipidaemia markers

675 Tendon xanthomata in the Achilles tendon. Minor fusiform swelling of the tendon will be missed unless a search is made in heterozygous **familial hypercholesterolaemia**.

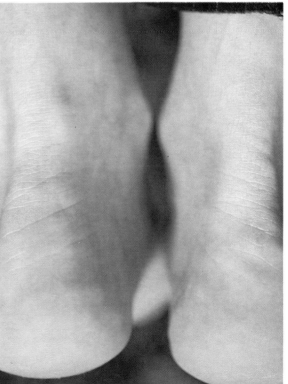

675

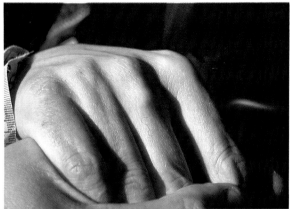

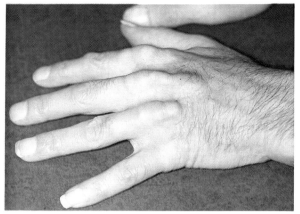

678

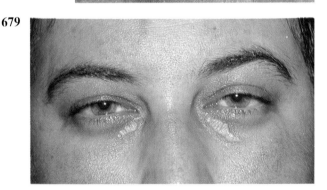

676 Tendon xanthomata in the extensor tendon over the base of the proximal phalanx middle finger of the same patient as in **675**.

677 Marked tendon xanthomata—familial hyper-cholesterolaemia.

678 Arcus cornealis. Though the deposit of lipid seen at the limbus of the eye and in the skin around the eyes is found in **familial hypercholesterolaemia**, it is not much help in making the diagnosis, being common in the elderly (but it may be more closely associated in the young).

679 Xanthelasma palpebrarum. These lesions, which occur in familial hypercholesterolaemia, should not be confused with epidermal cysts to which they bear a superficial resemblance. Like corneal arcus, they are not helpful as they may be absent in a heteroxygote for familial hyper-cholesterolaemia yet present in normal individuals. They are common in obese middle-aged females.[1]

679

[1] See Durrington, Paul. *Hyperlipidaemia*. Wright, 1989.

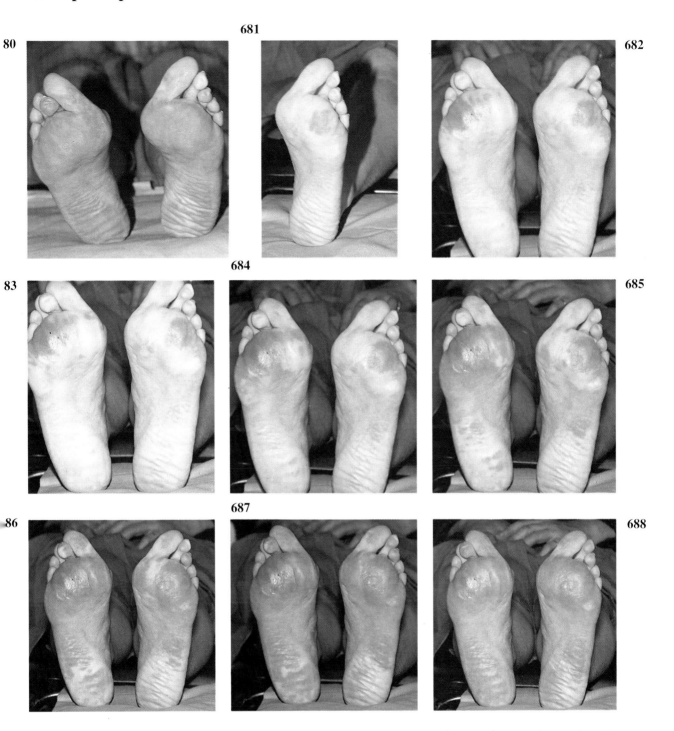

680–688 Raynaud's phenomenon of the feet. A woman aged 58 with systemic sclerosis and rheumatoid arthritis prior to exposure to cold (**680**) contrasts with the intense pallor of vasoconstriction (**681**) after she volunteered to walk around Fitzroy Square in London in open sandals in the winter! During rewarming (**682–687**) cyanosis developed as the capillaries and venules dilated and the blood became deoxygenated. The phenomenon is completed by the bright red colour of reactive hyperaemia (**688**). This physical sign is seen more frequently in the upper limb, and may affect only

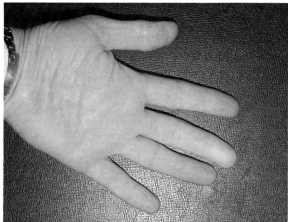

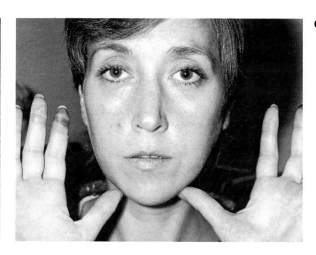

one digit (**689**), with the intense pallor, or may be bilateral and so severe as to cause gangrene (**690**). The ptosis on the side of the most severe ischaemic change was caused by cervical sympathectomy in an attempt to alleviate the vasospasm—a sympathetic nerve lesion with partial ptosis and a small pupil. There is over-reaction of the frontalis on the same side as the ptosis.

When no underlying disease is found, this is primary Raynaud's disease; when an underlying condition is present, it is a secondary phenomenon. Underlying disease may include occlusive arterial disease, connective tissue disorders such as progressive systemic sclerosis, rheumatoid arthritis,

and systemic lupus erythematosus—as well as being part of the CREST syndrome (Calcinosis, Raynaud's, Esophageal dysmotility, Sclerodactyly and Telangiectasia). It may precede these disorders by years.

It is also associated with minor repetitive trauma, and may be seen in the upper limb with neurogenic problems such as cervical rib and syringomyelia, which may result from irritation to the sympathetic nerve supply. Drugs such as ergotamine, and exposure to polyvinylchloride, may cause it, and it may be seen in patients taking beta-blocking agents as well as in states associated with cold agglutinins.

Circulatory problems related to temperature

Cold injury

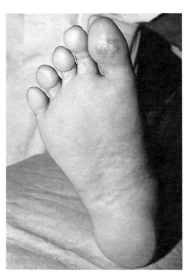

692

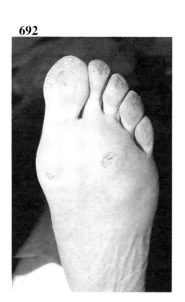

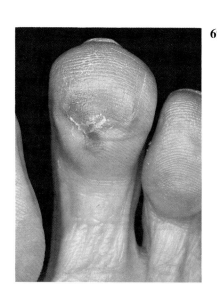

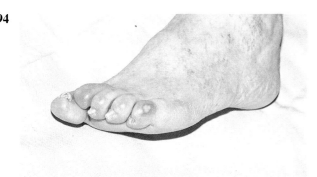

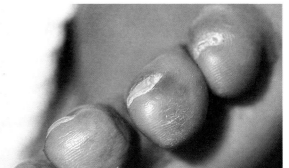

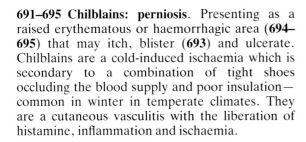

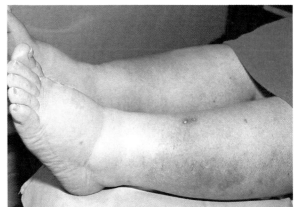

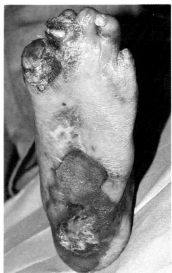

691–695 Chilblains: perniosis. Presenting as a raised erythematous or haemorrhagic area (**694–695**) that may itch, blister (**693**) and ulcerate. Chilblains are a cold-induced ischaemia which is secondary to a combination of tight shoes occluding the blood supply and poor insulation—common in winter in temperate climates. They are a cutaneous vasculitis with the liberation of histamine, inflammation and ischaemia.

695 A Kuwaiti girl aged 30 came to London in mid-January for a university term break. Shopping in sandals in Bond Street led to an itch and pain in the tips of her toes, so she bought a pair of furlined boots.

Perniosis may be caused by tight jeans and the insulation produced by fat thighs may lead to an ischaemic cold injury to the thigh, the skin becoming pink, blue and mottled (cutis marmorata). This change is seen in the legs of this fat female (**696**), where winter chilling has led to pink mottling. Lymphoedema is present.

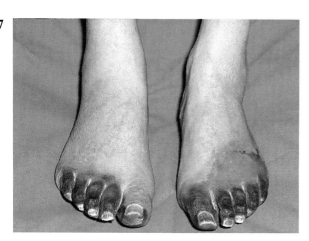

697 Severe frostbite—acute. Gangrene of all toes secondary to cold injury is seen in this alcoholic man who spent a November night on a bench on the Embankment in London, using newspapers to cover his trunk to keep warm. The frostbite was aggravated by an impaired arterial circulation. The line of demarcation with erythema can be seen on the right foot, in particular. The man lost some toes but retained good function.

698 Residual damage. The damaged frozen tissue simulates tissue damage produced by burns. Sensitivity to cold and pain on walking may remain for years.

699

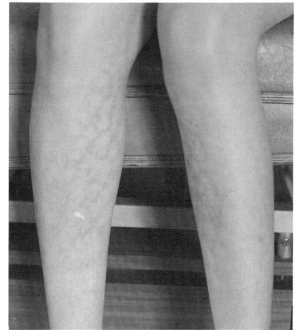

701

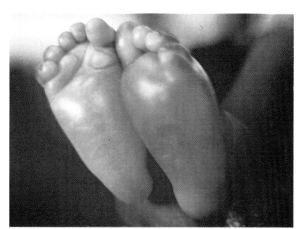

70

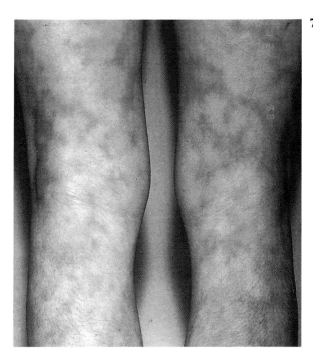

699 Legs: erythema ab igne. Seen in winter, especially in those whose legs are exposed and who huddle close to an open fire—from its distribution one may deduce the side of the fire on which the person sits! There is erythema with brown pigmentation related to degradation of haemoglobin in the skin. Removal from the heat will lead to slow clearing.

700 Legs: livedo reticularis. Cooled skin may become mottled; if it is chronic it may lead to permanent change. It is more common in vascular insufficiency.

701 Burnt feet. Burns of the feet may occur with falls into open fires. The question to be asked is what is the reason for the fall? It may be due to epilepsy, or to a febrile convulsion in a child. This child had fever and malaria; the burn was due to immersion of the feet in a cooking pot of oil.

Circulatory problems due to pressure

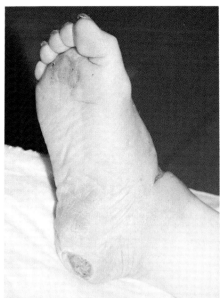

703

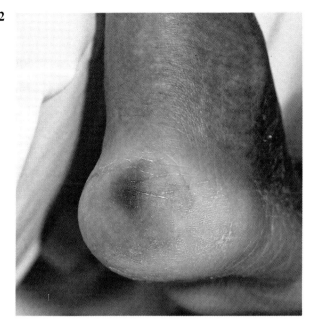

02

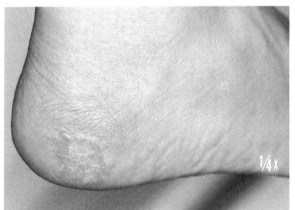

704

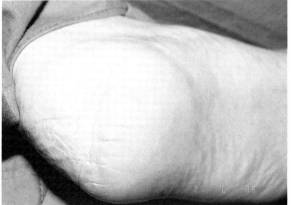

705

702 and 703 Simple pressure sores of the heel. Bed rest may lead to pressure sores. The prominence of the heel is at special risk during anaesthesia and illness. This man (**702**) developed an area of redness and central necrosis, which later separated leaving an ulcer which took three months to heal—though he was discharged from hospital following his coronary artery bypass within eight days. The morbidity was caused by a few hours' unrelieved pressure on the skin while in the intensive care unit.

The position of the ulcer in **703** must mean that the knee was flexed for a period, as the point of pressure has moved onto the sole. The man had been hit in the upper thigh by machine gun bullets while running to do his shopping (!) and the leg was put into traction with the knee bent. Unhappily, he also sloughed all the skin on the dorsum of the foot, where an intravenous infusion of a drug extravasated!

704 and 705 Pressure sore scars. This (**704**) is the remnant of a sore acquired in a few hours, perioperatively, the legs having been in an externally rotated position while the patient was unconscious. The scar does not encroach on the plantar surface, by contrast with **705**, which will always give trouble and may break down again.

706

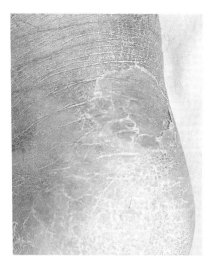

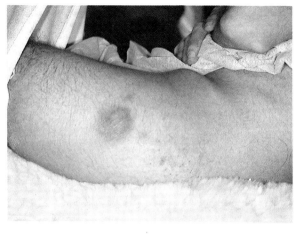

708

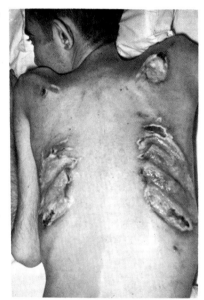

706 Shoe rub heel. The shoe which rubs at the top of the heel cup produces an ulcer over the Achilles tendon at a point higher than the bedsore. It is a potential cause of serious morbidity.

707 and 708 Bedsore greater trochanter. Twelve hours were sufficient to lead to a pressure blister over the bony prominence of the greater trochanter in this boy (**707**), who was severely ill with sickle cell anaemia complicated by salmonella osteomyelitis. If neglect is extreme, as in the paraplegic in **708**, then the sores will occur over any bony pressure point.

Circulatory problems due to blood disease

709

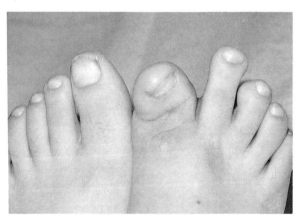

709 Sickle cell anaemia: the foot. The capillary bed seen through the nail is pale and the foot has pallor. It is crucial to appreciate the significance of the deformed phalanx of the great toe. This is the residuum of a bone infarct of sickle cell anaemia dactylitis earlier in childhood, and should alert one to the diagnosis.

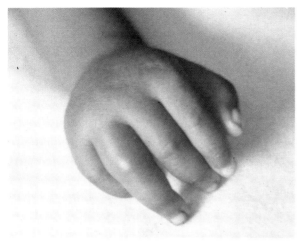

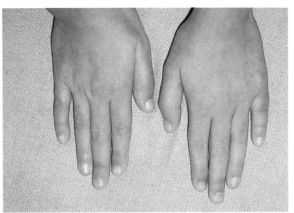

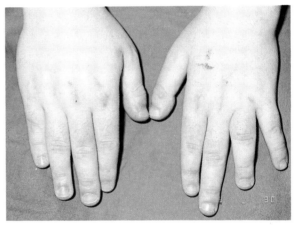

710–712 Sickle cell acute dactylitis. The acute pain and swelling of a bone crisis in the ring finger will lead to infarction and the appearance of the hand in **711**, where a short proximal phalanx has resulted. This should be differentiated from the short metacarpal seen in the bone disease of pseudohypoparathyroidism (**712**).

Multifactorial problems in gravitational ulcers

When venous insufficiency is the predominant factor the increased capillary pressure leads to increased permeability, and the migration of proteins and red cells into the tissue—which accounts for the brown pigmentation of haemosiderin staining and further fibrosis.

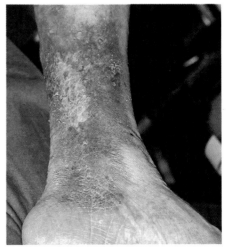

713 Brown pigmentation of the lower third of the leg. Medial pigmentation of venous insufficiency occurs. A scar from stripping of the long saphenous vein, and dry scales of skin, are present.

714

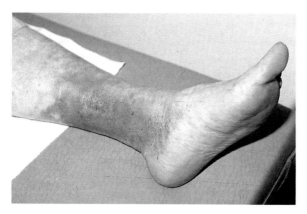

716

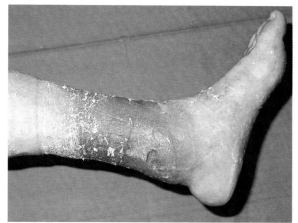

717

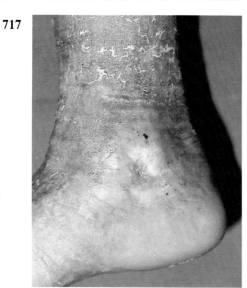

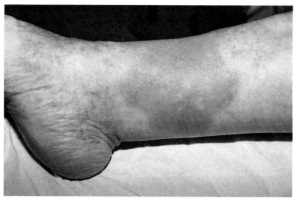

714 Brown pigmentation of varicose eczema leg. Haemosiderin deposition and tethering of the skin from fibrosis on the medial aspect of the leg in chronic venous insufficiency.

715 A red area on the lower third of a leg with eczema, on a Cypriot machinist aged 40. The recurrent inflammation and subsequent fibrosis lead to tethering of the skin, which is seen in profile along the upper border. Haemosiderin pigment is seen.

716 Eczema and punched out ulcer. An elderly man with an immobile ischaemic foot with extensive pigmentation due to venous insufficiency and an indolent ulcer. Ischaemia complicates the venous insufficiency.

717 A healing ulcer around internal malleous. The ulcer has healed after the application of supportive bandaging from toe to knee.

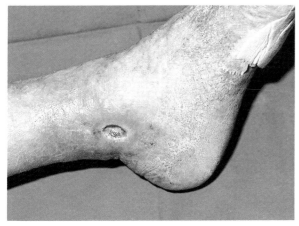

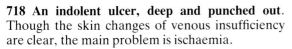

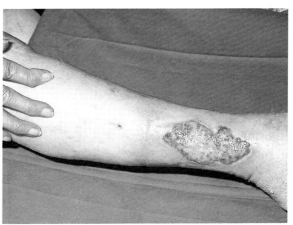

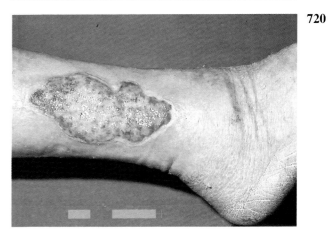

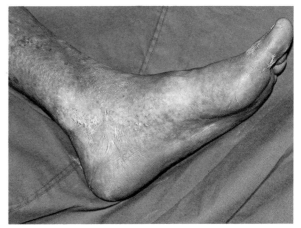

718 An indolent ulcer, deep and punched out. Though the skin changes of venous insufficiency are clear, the main problem is ischaemia.

719 and 720 A long-standing gravitational ulcer. Squamous carcinomatous change may occur in chronic ulcers. The exuberant appearance of the base of this ulcer is suggestive of neoplastic change (**719**). The hand (**720**) shows osteoarthritic stigmata in the index finger (Heberden's node), and the scar of knee joint replacement surgery can also be seen. That operation was complicated by venous thrombosis and is an important factor in chronicity of the ulcer.

721 A leg with a healed ulcer. The leg is ischaemic, with venous stasis. The healed ulcer was originally related to minor trauma; healing was prolonged, and the leg remains at risk if it is injured again.

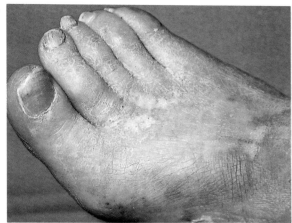

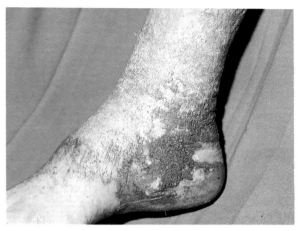

724

725

722 Atrophie blanche. The appearance at the base of the 2nd and 3rd toes is due to the obliteration of capillaries in the upper dermis causing sclerosis. Residual vessels are attenuated and liable to thrombosis with consequent ulceration. This may be seen in gravitational stasis and venous obstruction, as well as in many vasculitides.

723 and 724 Lymphoedema verrucosa.[2] See page 131.

725 A gravitational ulcer on the heel, in a case of secondary lymphoedema. The verrucous change of lymphoedema.

Not all leg ulcers are gravitational. An assessment of the venous and ischaemic components must be made. Atypical ulcers may be related to blood disease—sickle cell anaemia, syphilis, yaws, or pyoderma gangrenosum—as well as to dermatitis artefacta, or to a vasculitis (as in rheumatoid arthritis).

[2]Lymphoedema. *Lancet*, March 22, 1986.

12 The foot in neurological disease

What appearances in the lower limb and foot suggest neurological disease?

- In motion: gait
- At rest: muscle bulk
  posture
  skin changes

Damage to the upper motor neurone may be appreciated in subtle ways by the patient long before any change in appearance or physical sign is present.

Complaints of scuffing the toe or tripping over cracks, or of difficulty in climbing stairs from hip flexor weakness, should be treated with diligent analysis and follow up. When the patient steps off a kerb and places the plantar-flexed toe to the ground, clonus may occur as the foot is dorsiflexed and takes the weight of the upper body—and be described in graphic manner! The appearance of the full hemiplegic or paraplegic gait will come much later. A spastic paraparesis with rigid limbs, adducted and plantar flexed, leads to a gait whose appearance, with the legs dragged past one another—suggests that the patient will topple forwards; the spastic hemiplegic gait—a circumduction and dragging of one limb—may wear the toe of the shoe.

In motion

Gait—circumducting hemiplegic

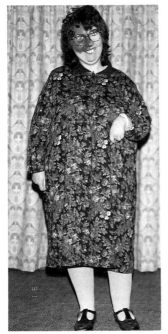

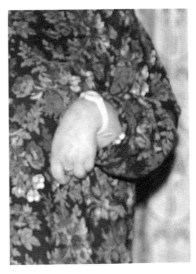

726 Hemiplegic posture. The left arm is adducted, flexed at the elbow, while the hand is clenched and smaller than the right (retarded growth). The left leg is not carrying weight in this position of ease, and is fatter as the calf pump mechanism works less efficiently. The leg is spastic and so is circumducted on walking. The facial birthmark and glass eye are a clue to the aetiology.[1]

[1]Intra-cranial haemangioma in the Sturge–Weber syndrome.

727 Hemiplegic's shoe. The gait leads to wear on the tip and medial aspect of the sole of the shoe as the upper motor-neurone (umn) lesion causes dragging of the affected leg, abducting it in an arc with the toe scraping the floor. The problem is due to weak hip flexion, knee flexion, dorsiflexion eversion of the foot—those muscle groups that are affected earliest by upper motor neurone weakness.

Where else to look
728 Hemiplegic arm and hand posture. The fist is clenched, and the arm flexed at the elbow and adducted to the body.

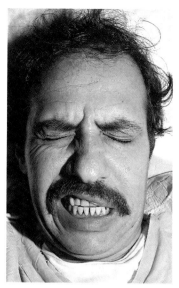

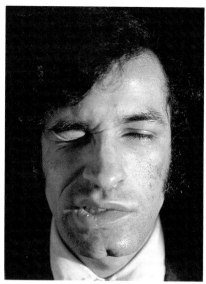

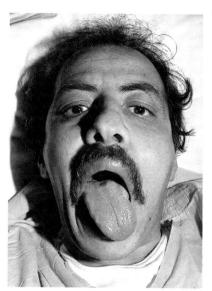

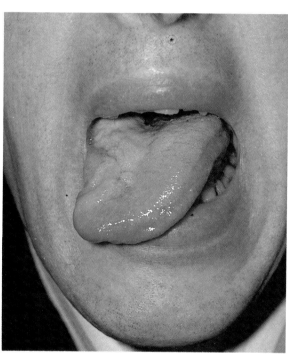

729 Upper motor neurone lesion of the 7th nerve palsy of the face. The cerebral hemisphere has most influence over the contralateral lower face: the upper face and eyelids concerned with reflex protection are innervated from both sides. This man has had a right cerebrovascular accident (CVA), and experiences weakness in the lower face on the left when asked to show the teeth and screw up the eyes. The weakness of the upper face is much less marked because of the bilateral supranuclear connections.

730 Lower motor neurone palsy of the face — differential diagnosis. By contrast with **729**, a *lower* motor-neurone lesion affects the whole face. This man is performing the same action as depicted in **729**, and can screw up the eye and show the teeth on the normal side with weakness of all the face on the left.

731 Upper motor neurone lesion of the 12th nerve: **effect on the tongue**. A CVA leading to an upper motor-neurone lesion on the left will lead to weakness of the tongue, which will deviate to the side of the weakness as the strong side pushes it across. Wasting is minimal, by contrast to a lower motor-neurone lesion (**732**). This man has a neuroma in the jugular foramen which has compressed the nerve.

The plantar response

733–734 The extensor plantar response — the Babinsky* response. The sign of an upper motor-neurone lesion. Suspect it when testing the tone by rolling the leg (external/internal rotation at the hip). Elicit it with a blunt pointed object — for example, a key (**733**) — by stroking the lateral border of the foot firmly (warn the patient!): watch closely. In an early lesion, the up-going toe (**734**) may appear only once or twice, and then you will be in the doubtful area of 'the plantars are equivocal'! The extension of the great toe may be accompanied by fanning of the lesser toes. It is the initial movement that is crucial, and this must be distinguished from the movement of withdrawal from an unpleasant stimulus. The extensor plantar response means there is a lesion of the pyramidal tract.

*Joseph François Felix Babinsky, 1857–1932

734

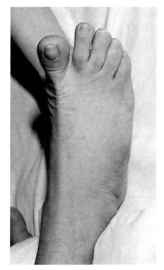

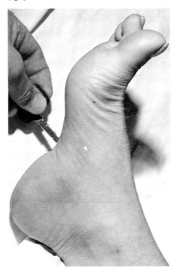

733

During walking the two feet are on the ground for a very short time. In small vessel cerebro-vascular disease the duration is increased and the steps become smaller—*marche aux petit pas*. Lack of confidence, with a fear of falling, may be a further reason for a shuffle gait, with the soles brushing the ground—which may make tripping over paving stones more possible. The rigidity of extrapyramidal disease may lead to a loss of arm swing, a restricted gait, and small steps, with an appearance of hurrying to keep one's centre of gravity within the area of the feet, as the arms are not used to maintain balance. A diagnosis may be made by the sound of the steps if the rhythm is noted.

736

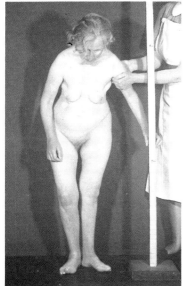

735

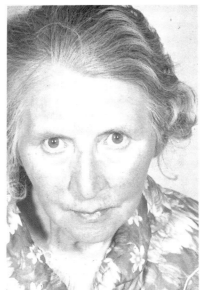

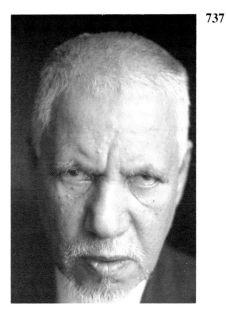

737

Festinant Parkinsonian gait

735 Parkinson's disease.* The gait is accompanied by a flexed position of the neck, as if an invisible pillow propped it forward, and the gaze is seen from beneath the eyebrows. The arm is flexed and adducted, and the normal arm swing is lost. The steps are small with a poverty of movement.

*James Parkinson, British physician, 1755–1824, described 1817.

736 and 737 Parkinsonian facies. The neck flexion leads to a gaze that appears to emanate from directly beneath the eyebrows, and which is combined with a blank facial visage due to a paucity of facial movement—which may well contrast with the active anguished mind within! Rigidity is seen in the sternomastoids, which stand out like bowstrings!

738

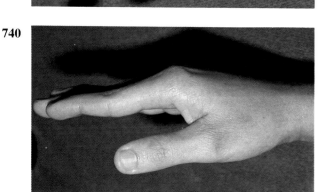

With very many thanks + best wi-
-h the New Year

Yrs sincerely,
Russell. --- 1986

Yrs sincerely
Russell. --- 1984

Yrs sincerely,
Russell --- 1983

Regards,
Russell. --- 1978

Regards,
Russell. --- 1973

739

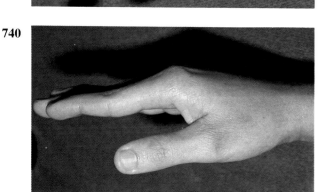

740

741

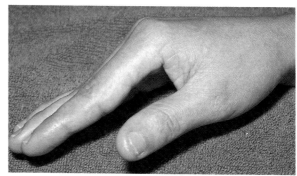

738 Parkinsonian writing. Over 13 years the signature of this patient has changed, the words becoming smaller and the letters less rounded, as the limb has become rigid and limited in its generosity of smooth movement. The letters are jerky, and reflect the diminished control over tremor.

739–741 Parkinsonian tremor of the hand. The tremor of Parkinson's disease is seen first at rest and can be inhibited by movement; more severe disease may be associated with tremor on action. At rest, tremor may be due to anxiety, thyrotoxicosis, alcohol, or benign essential tremor, as well as to dopamine deficiency disease. On movement, it occurs in Parkinson's disease, essential tremor, and cerebellar disease. The characteristic movement can be seen in these three illustrations of a hand flexing at the metacarpophalangeal joints, and extending at the wrist at a frequency of 1–3 cycles/sec. —leading to the pill rolling description. Anxiety aggravates the condition.

High-stepping/stamping gait, heard or seen

This suggests a sensory proprioceptive disorder or a foot drop from muscular weakness. The gait of peripheral muscle weakness can be heard as the feet slap on the floor from foot drop. An ataxic gait combined with an excessive lift occurs from loss of proprioceptive information and is seen in posterior column disease.

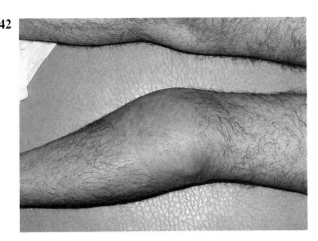

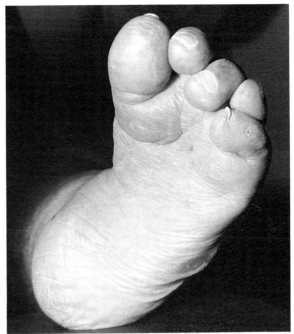

742 A neuropathic knee joint—tabes dorsalis. An unsteady gait with high steps, poor balance in the dark, and a tendency to fall when washing the face: all reflect proprioceptive loss. The failure of deep pain sensation leads to excessive strains and a painless joint with an abnormal range of movement.

743 Polio in childhood—foot drop. The lower motor weakness has led to an inability to dorsiflex and evert the foot. To clear the ground the leg is lifted higher and a callus appears on the lateral part of the foot. A unilateral foot drop may be due to a lesion of the motor cortex foot area, of the L5 root by pressure from a prolapsed disc, or of the common peroneal nerve which will supply the anterior compartment of the leg. It may be damaged at the fibula neck, by an injection in the buttock, or by a hip fracture or dislocation. There may be sensory loss over the lateral foot, but not if the cause of the foot drop is polio.

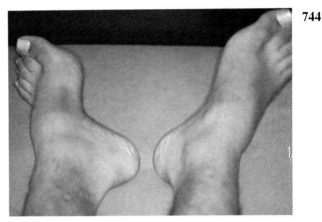

744 Polio pes cavus. A lone lower motor neurone weakness without sensory loss, the foot changing because of the muscle imbalance.

745 and 746 Polio in childhood—foot drop and cavus foot. The weight of the short flaccid leg is taken on the lateral forefoot because of a foot drop due to a weakness of the tibialis anterior.

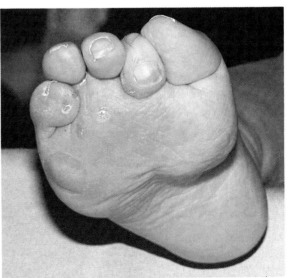

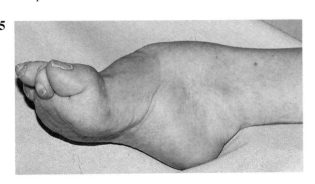

747

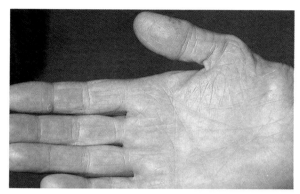

74

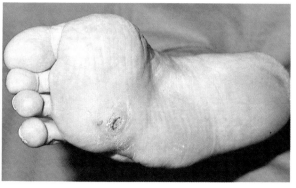

749

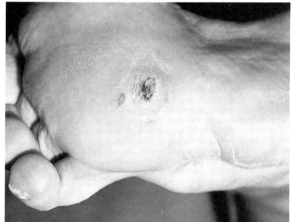

747 Polio wasting. Wasting may be asymmetrical and localised, depending on the random nature of the anterior horn cell invasion. The thenar eminence and particularly abductor pollicis brevis is affected. There is a verruca on the index finger.

748-750 Polio: iatrogenic sensory loss and a neuropathic ulcer. Foot drop due to polio. Unusually, a neuropathic ulcer is present, but the sensory loss is iatrogenic. The scar (**749**) of a tendon transplant operation has cut the sensory nerves and led to an ulcer over the area that bears weight. Note the absence of sweating over the anaesthetic area (**750**).

750

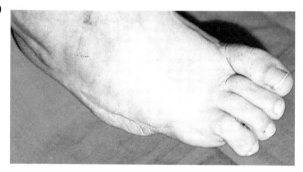

A limp or an uneven gait

A limp or an uneven gait may be the result of pain, disparity in limb length, or muscle weakness.

751

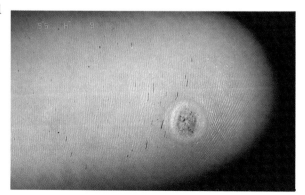

An antalgic gait due to pain

751 Verruca of the sole of the foot. A viral wart on the sole of the foot is a common cause of a painful limp. Dermal ridges are absent and thrombosed vessels in the papillae show as dots.

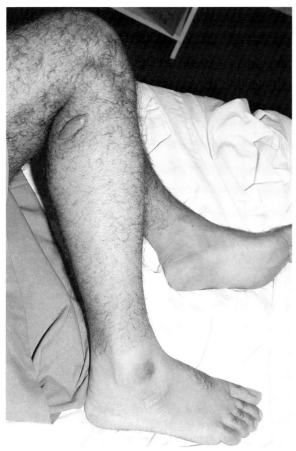

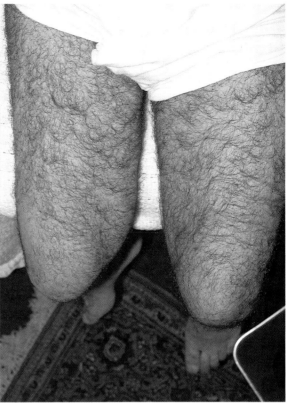

752 Cautery of the leg. Pain in the lower back which radiates down the leg may be caused by pressure on a nerve root. Weakness may lead to a limp. This man had L 5 root pain distributed down the lateral leg to the foot: a healer had treated it with counter-irritation in the form of the cautery. The keloid scar at the proximal end of the dermatome suggests a burn and gives a clue to the length of the history. The majority of backaches will clear in six months, ensuring that this form of treatment will have success and potentiate its use!

Gait due to weakness

753 and 754 Polio limb and shortening. The femur is short (**753**), and so is the tibia (**754**). There is global muscle wasting with a flaccid foot drop.

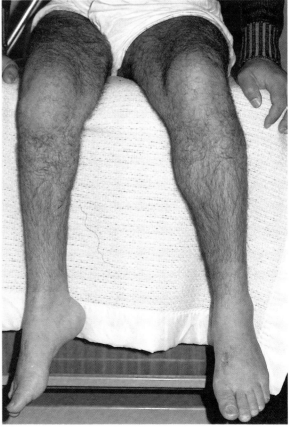

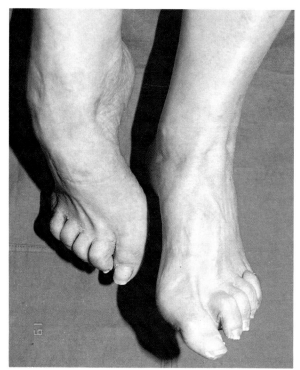

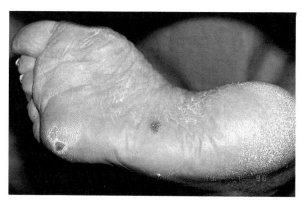

Gait due to shortening

755 and 756 Foot drop and shortening. A spinster aged 65 had a hip joint replacement. Subsequent dislocation of the prosthesis posteriorly damaged the common peroneal component of the sciatic nerve, leading to foot drop (**755**) with the weight taken on the lateral border over the 5th metatarsal (mt) head. The two longitudinal skin creases on the forefoot (**756**) indicate rotational movement on the pivotal point.

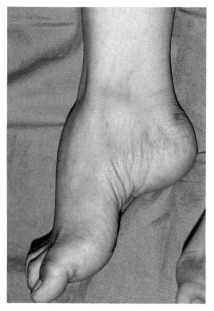

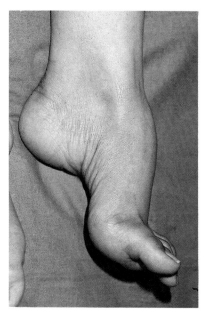

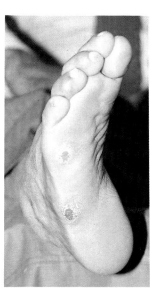

757 and 758 Bilateral foot drop in polio. Polio occurred in adolescence and has produced bilateral foot drop secondary to weakness of the dorsiflexors of the ankle.

759 Right leg and foot, old polio. A slim Asian man aged 38 had polio with residual peroneal weakness at the age of 11 years. His weight is borne sequentially from the base of the 5th mt to the 5th head and on push off on the lateral side of the 4th toe.

At rest

Observe: muscle bulk

- Generalised disuse atrophy of the limb muscles may occur in an upper motor neurone lesion
- Generalised proximal muscle wasting—polymyositis or endocrinopathy
- Isolated anterior thigh wasting in a femoral nerve neuropathy—diabetic amyotrophy
- Localised muscle wasting ceasing half way up leg—Charcot Marie Tooth* neuropathy

- Unilateral loss of muscle bulk—old polio
- Loss confined to one muscle group—damage to lateral peroneal nerve

and

- Fasciculation—motor neurone disease

Observe: posture

60

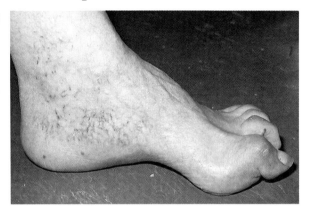

761

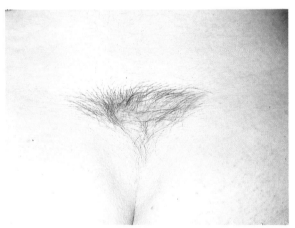

762

760 Pes cavus *and* retracted toes. Pes cavus describes a foot with an exaggerated longitudinal arch. It may be either a lone feature with potential painful problems, or a pointer to diagnosis—in a patient or the family—of a neurological disorder.

In the inherited peripheral neuropathies such as peroneal muscular atrophy, hypertrophic peripheral neuropathy and Friedreich's ataxia (which has a peripheral neuropathic component), pes cavus may occur in affected or unaffected family members.

761 Retracted toes alone. The intrinsic muscles are not stabilising the metatarsophalangeal (mtp) joints and the extensor muscles cause hyperextension at these joints. The condition may occur in the weakness of motor neurone disease.

Neurological conditions associated with pes cavus

Spinal dysraphism in its most florid form of incomplete closure of the vertebral canal may be associated with a similar anomaly of the spinal cord. Minor forms may be associated with intraspinal (IS) abnormalities and neurological changes.

762 Spina bifida occulta. If symptoms are present there may be some external physical sign. A tuft of hair alone or in association with an area of atrophic skin as can be seen overlying the sacrum at the apex of the natal cleft. The clue may be a naevus or lipoma over the lesion.

*Jean Martin Charcot, French neurologist, 1825–1893.
Howard Henry Tooth, English neurologist, 1856–1925, described 1886.

763

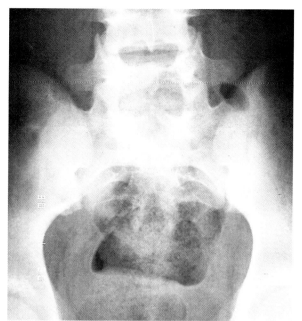

764

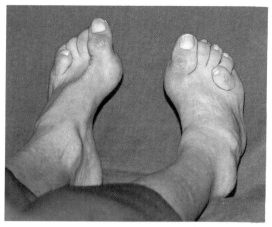

765

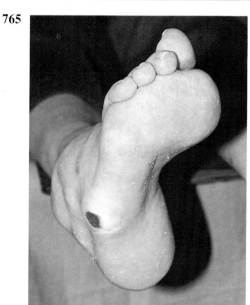

763 An X-ray: spina bifida occulta. The defect in the vertebral arch is seen. It may be quite asymptomatic or associated with a syndrome of pes cavus and a short leg and neurological deficit. Sphincter disturbances with a neuropathic bladder or faecal incontinence may occur and may only present in later life. The differential diagnosis of spinal dysraphism will include other causes of pes cavus.

764 and 765 Spina bifida feet. A man aged 49 with spina bifida is nevertheless still able to support himself by working full time. He wears surgical shoes with suitable insoles. There is a neuropathic ulcer over the base of the 5th mt.

766 Spina bifida and pes cavus. A man aged 49 with spina bifida and resulting pes cavus. On the right, overloading of the 2nd mt head led to pain and its removal 16 years earlier. The consequent transfer overload to the 3rd mt head (arrow) causes similar pain.

766

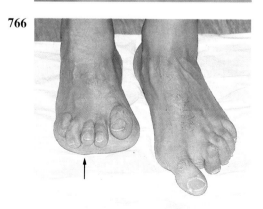

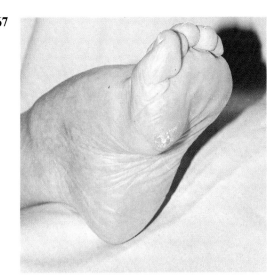

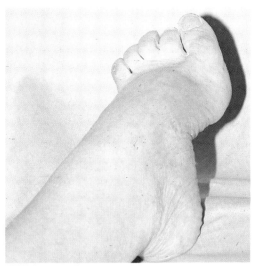

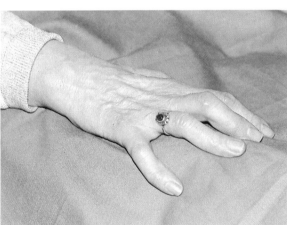

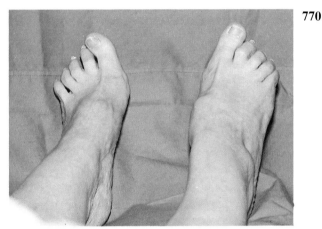

767 and 768 Talipes equino varus. By contrast with **766**, a mobile plantar-flexed foot with humping of the tarsus. The position of the skin creases and the area of callus over the 1st mtp joint indicate the movement and loading on weight bearing.

- **Muscle weakness**
  - Lower motor neurone palsy: *polio*
  - Muscle disorder, *Charcot-Marie Tooth, Friedreich's ataxia*
  - Anterior horn cell dysfunction: *motor neurone disease* (look for claw toes and small muscle wasting
- **Neuropathy**
  - Small muscle wasting, thigh wasting: *Diabetes*.

769 and 770 Motor neurone disease. A woman aged 69 with small muscle wasting of the hand (**769**), making small fine movements difficult. The intrinsic muscles of the feet are also affected, causing instability and deformity of the forefeet (**770**).

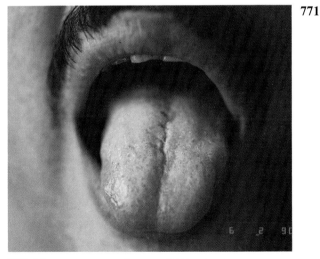

771 Motor neurone disease. Difficulty in swallowing and speech due to the bulbar involvement is reflected in the small fasciculating tongue in this Saudi Arabian aged 40.

Skin change

Signs suggesting neuropathy

- **Ulcers**   anaesthetic feet, diabetes (q.v.) and leprosy
- **Callus**   diabetes
- **Oedema**   and volume increase, feet swollen, neurofibromatosis
- **Muscle wasting**

772

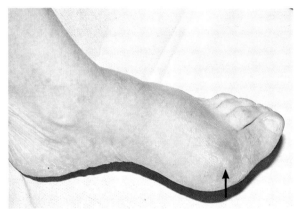

773

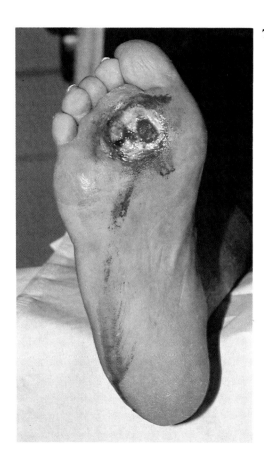

774

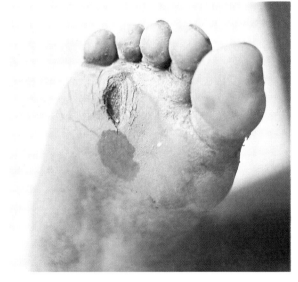

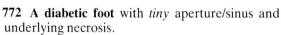

772 A diabetic foot with *tiny* aperture/sinus and underlying necrosis.

773 A diabetic ulcer juicily infected. Both this and the example in **772** may occur in diabetes and are often complicated by an underlying neuropathy.

774 Leprosy: a dry perforating ulcer. A trophic ulcer related to sensory loss may be seen in neuropathic conditions such as tuberculoid leprosy or tabes dorsalis. Note that there is no toe retraction and the foot is heavily calloused from walking barefoot. In diabetes, ulcers are more common over the 1st and 5th mt heads, but can occur over any mt head which is exposed to extra loading when the retracted toes exacerbate the overload. This foot does not feel pain but there is no evidence of overloading.

75

777

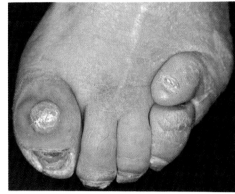

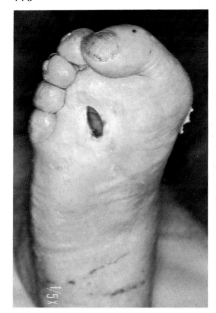

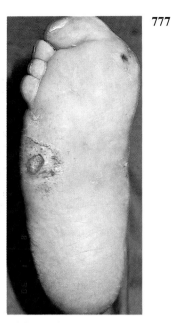

775–777 Tuberculoid leprosy. The *essential* problem is loss of pain sensation, leading to repeated trauma as well as motor weakness and consequent deformity. Lack of pain leads to destruction and motor loss to deformity. The scar on the dorsum (**775**) is from a tendon transplant operation. Autonomic denervation leads to dry and atrophic skin. There is callus over the dorsum of the great toe but without underlying break-down. The diabetic neuropathic foot has additional ischaemic/infective components which change the time scale of healing or cause a more rapid aggressive destructive breakdown. This is empha-sised by the change in sole view (**776–777**) after half a decade of protective chiropodial care.

778 Leprosy: a neck with thickened nerves. Thickened nerves may be seen in the posterior triangle of the neck, with a palpable and visible greater auricular nerve. In the leg the lateral popliteal nerve may be palpable as it winds around the neck of the fibula. The differential diagnosis of thickened nerves includes the inherited neuro-pathies such as peroneal muscular atrophy, infiltrations with amyloid or local neuromata, and the effect of trauma.

778

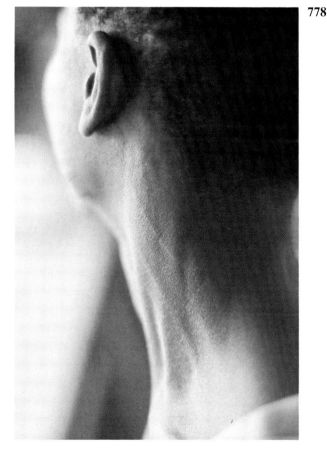

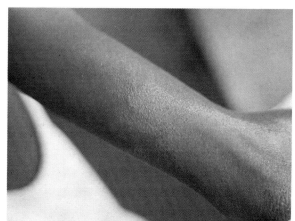

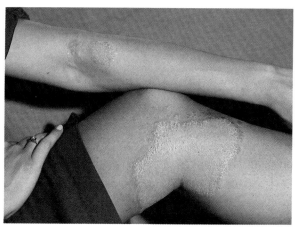

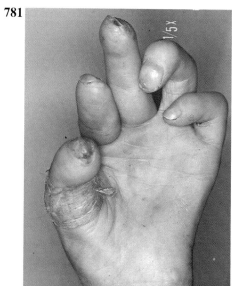

78

779 Leprosy: the skin of the arm. The skin lesions run in a spectrum from the diffuse infiltration of lepromatous leprosy to the raised-pebbled and well-defined scaly patch with an anaesthetic centre of major tuberculoid leprosy. Between the two, borderline leprosy may present as a pale rough anaesthetic patch—but be less circumscribed as it is not being contained.

780 Leprosy: the leg. Major tuberculoid leprosy must be distinguished from other conditions. Biopsy of this lesion showed granulomata, and a suggested diagnosis of sarcoidosis was discarded when the anaesthetic skin over the plaque on the leg was demonstrated.

781 Leprosy: the simian hand. The motor loss leads to weakness and wasting with deformity—flat thenar eminence due to median palsy and hypothenar flattening due to ulnar palsy. The sensory loss leads to trophic changes from recurrent trauma.

782 Lepromatous leprosy: facies. The skin is thickened, especially over the ears—which show nodules—and over the eyebrows, where there is hair loss. The skin of the nose and lips is infiltrated. The thick skin develops folds, until the leonine appearance is complete.

783–786 Neurofibromatosis, type 1 NF.[1]

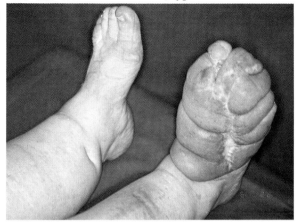

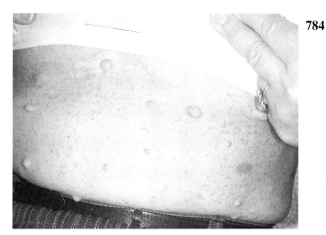

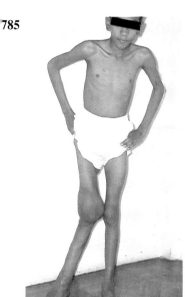

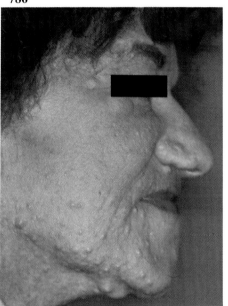

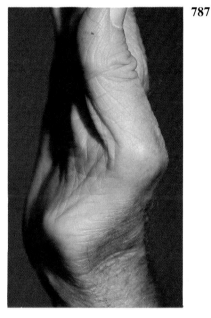

783 Plexiform neurofibroma. The presence of more than half a dozen café au lait pigmented patches on the body should raise the question of neurofibromatosis. If subcutaneous neurofibromata are found or the presence of a plexiform neurofibroma or iris nodules noted then the diagnosis of Type 1 NF is clear.

784 Abdomen with café au lait spots and multiple neurofibromata.

785 Café au lait spots on the trunk and a neuropathic joint. The swollen knee joint is due to the damage inflicted on the nerve roots in the lumbar area by a dumbell tumour compressing the root in the intervertebral foramen.

786 Subcutaneous nodules may not be present at birth but may appear in childhood. A family history of this autosomal dominant disorder may not be obtained as new cases are often due to mutation. Its recognition may help other members of the family, particularly type 2 NF when sparse cutaneous manifestations may be present yet the patient may have bilateral acoustic neuromata.

787 Wasting of the thumb. Don't forget that muscle wasting can be due to local causes such as painful arthritis or reflect lower motor neurone disease in a peripheral neuropathy, nerve compression, spinal root lesions or anterior horn cell pathology.

[1]Clinico-pathological Conference, *New Eng. J. Med.*, April 13, 1989 (type i neurofibromatosis).

13 The foot and nails in dermatology

The quality of the skin changes with ageing.

788 The young foot. The bloom of youth is seen in the foot as everywhere else! Young feet are moist, the tissues elastic, they may smell due to bacterial decomposition of the sweat, are well endowed with fibro-fatty padding, and usually have little shoe moulding.

789 The old foot. The skin is dry and thin, with the loss of elasticity and fibro-fatty padding. The interface with the environment may be reflected in damage from the sun, heat, cold or mechanical trauma, which may delay healing. There may be evidence of recurrent mechanical trauma and the effects of shoe moulding.

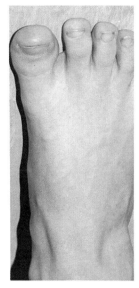
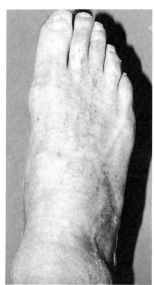

Keratinisation and its associations

Plantar hyperkeratosis may be inherited in an autosomal dominant fashion as diffuse palmar plantar keratoderma or tylosis, when it is diffuse, smooth and uniform, with a tendency to fissuring. Much is made of the association with oesophageal malignancy.

790

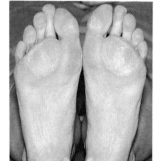

791

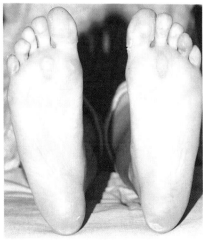

792

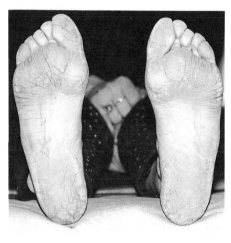

790 Hyperkeratosis familial. The tendency may occur in families, this woman having hyperkeratotic soles, as did three siblings and her son.

791 Hyperkeratotic soles. This condition began at the age of five years in both mother and (seen here) daughter.

792 Hyperkeratosis in a 43-year-old, again from the age of five. One son is affected.

793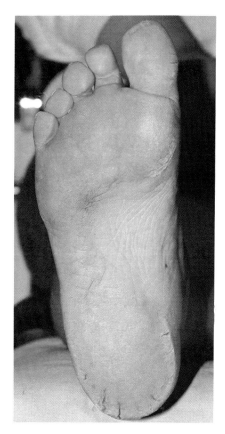

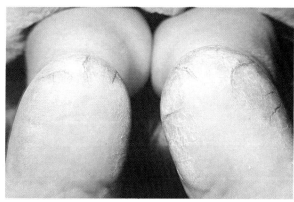
79

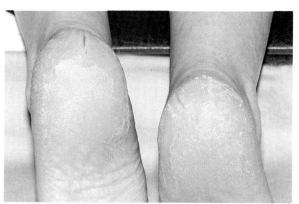
79

793 Heel fissures. Hyperkeratotic soles are prone to fissure development. These in a woman aged 41 have been present for ten years.

794 and 795 Congenital hyperkeratosis. Fissures have developed at the heel and extend deeply into the tissues, remaining (**795**) after the hardened skin has been pared away.

796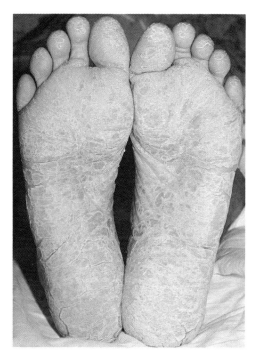

796 Drug-induced hyperkeratosis (practolol). Beta adrenoreceptor blocking agents may induce lichenoid or psoriasiform rashes. This reaction occurred in a woman on practolol who developed the oculocutaneous syndrome with dry eyes, skin rashes, these feet, and a fibrinous peritonitis.

Friction and the skin

Man cannot function without friction between himself and his environment. Low-intensity friction will induce hyperkeratosis, leading to corns, calluses and lichenification and pigmentation. High-intensity sudden friction leads to blister formation. Friction is reduced by dry skin and increased when it is moist—if friction is intermittent then adaptation can take place and calluses form. Ageing skin is drier than the young variety (licking the finger to turn the page is more frequent as one approaches middle age!). Postural friction leads to a pressure dermatitis and the production of local callosities—hyperkeratinisation induced by recurrent friction and corns—over bony prominences. Callosities and corns may be occupational, due to habits, clothing, or weight bearing on the feet in association with abnormal mechanical stresses (when they must be differentiated from warts).

Keratinisation due to friction: deductions to be made

797

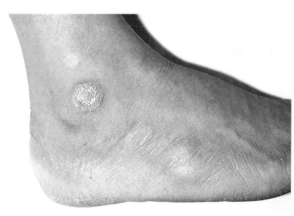

797 and 798 Callus on the ankle, related to sitting. In cultures where sitting on the floor is commonplace, calluses may be seen on the lateral aspect of the ankle—particularly in the devout Moslem.

798

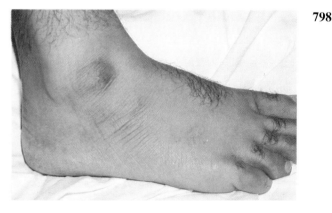

799

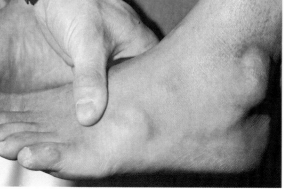

799 Callus on the ankle . . . and with a gouty tophus! The callus on the ankle is due to the friction involved in squatting on the floor, but the second lump on the lateral aspect of the foot has none of the surface keratinisation of a pressure dermatitis and is in fact a subcutaneous gouty tophus.

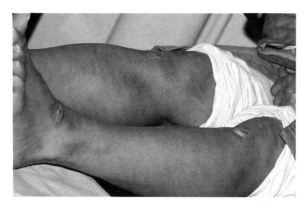

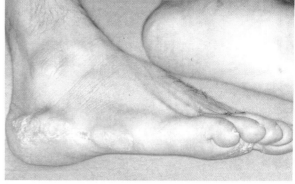

800 Callus on the anterior foot and knees. When the foot is hyperextended at the ankle, in the squatting position of prayer—the subject is a Moslem—the callus will be on the anterior aspect of one foot and on the skin overlying the tibial tubercle.

801 and 802 Prayer nodules. Intermittent friction against the ground leads to adaptive lichenification, pigmentation, and callus formation. Seen in men only, as the female covers her forehead when praying. It fades when illness prevents prayer, and is proportional to the frequency of devotions. The forehead illustrated (**802**) is of a sheikh (Muslim leader) of a mosque. The presence of nodules might lead to consideration of dose schedules and drug half lives during the fasting month of Ramadan, when food and drink or drugs can be taken only during the hours between sunset and sunrise.

802

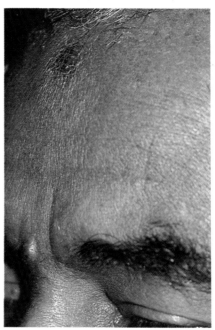

803

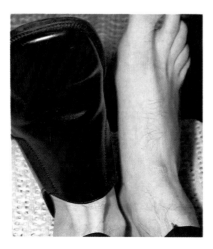

80

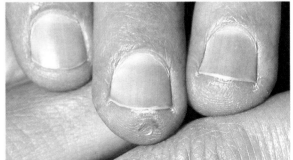

803 Callus on the foot of a chauffeur. The recurrent dorsal and plantar flexion at the ankle required to depress the clutch and brake pedals leads to calluses over the tendon of tibialis anterior where it rubs against the high-cut throat of the shoe upper.

804 A guitar player's fingers. The pressure exerted on a string of the instrument by the tip of the middle finger as it shortens the vibrating length can lead to hyperkeratosis.

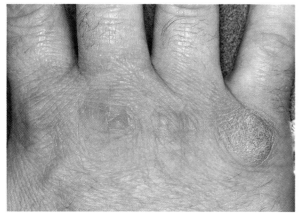

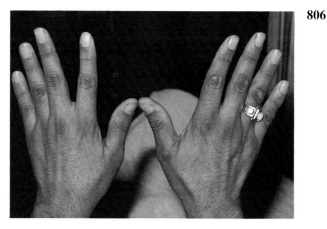

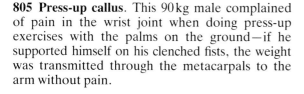

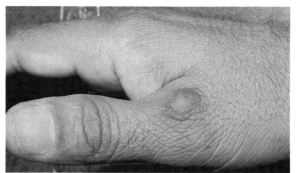

805 Press-up callus. This 90 kg male complained of pain in the wrist joint when doing press-up exercises with the palms on the ground—if he supported himself on his clenched fists, the weight was transmitted through the metacarpals to the arm without pain.

806 and 807 The Indian tailor's fingers. Callosities from cutting out suit patterns with scissors have developed over the metacarpophalangeal joint of the thumb and the proximal intraphalangeal joint of the ring finger of his right hand.

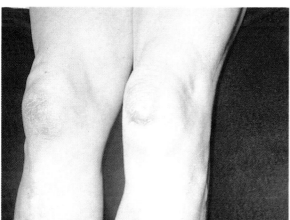

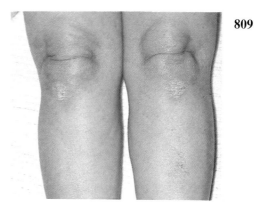

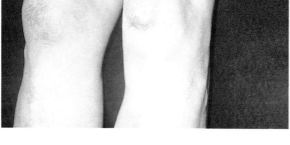

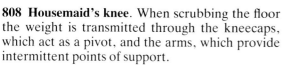

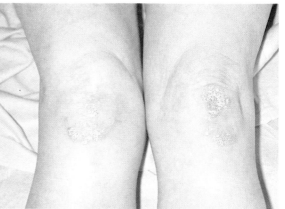

808 Housemaid's knee. When scrubbing the floor the weight is transmitted through the kneecaps, which act as a pivot, and the arms, which provide intermittent points of support.

809 and 810 Clergyman's knee. The tibial tubercle takes the pressure in recurrent kneeling, whereas the plaque of psoriasis (**810**) covers the tubercle and the adjacent skin.

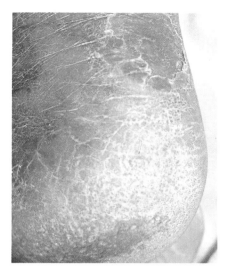

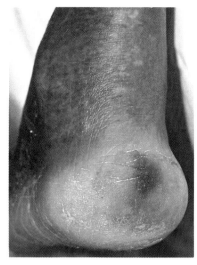

811 and 812 Shoe rub heel. Intense friction leads to blister formation —shoe rub—on the heel, at a site adjacent to the top of the heel of the shoe. By contrast, the pressure point when lying in bed (**812**) is the part of the heel where bedsores occur.

Inflammation of the skin: classical presentations

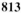

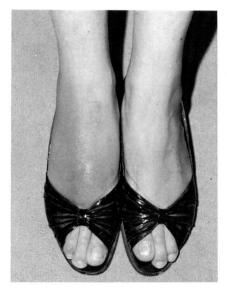

813 Erysipelas. A typical story: this riding instructress developed high fever, headache and rigors, and noted an ache in her right groin. The next day, a pink—and later, red—swollen area was seen over the dorsum of the foot. She felt a tender lump in the groin, and over the next week the red area spread—by the time she was seen, it was already subsiding. In the meantime, she had been thought to have had a virus, a skin allergy, an inguinal hernia and trauma from a horse. This is erysipelas, which is usually seen on the face or limbs, and is caused by a group A streptococcus spreading in the cutaneous lymphatics.

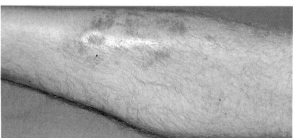

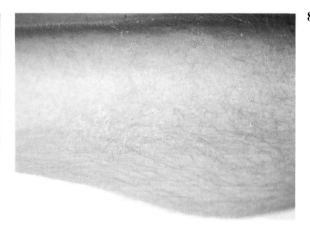

814 and 815 Erysipelas leg. This physician became febrile and then felt some pain in the leg, a groin gland, and then noted the changes seen in **814**. The edge is scarlet, oedematous, and pits on pressure; central clearing of the lesion occurs. It recurred a year later. As it heals, desquamation is seen (**815**).

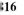

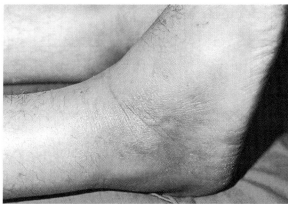

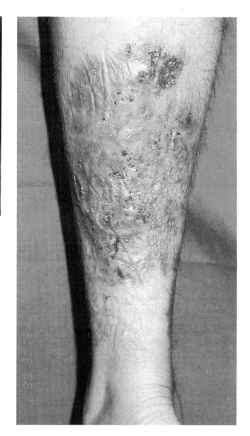

816 Recurrent erysipelas. Subcutaneous fibrosis will occur if the condition is recurrent, when the skin will feel tethered and immobile. The condition is best appreciated if the skin is pinched up between finger and thumb (see page 131).

817 and 818 Pyoderma gangrenosum. A Greek ship's captain presented with an ulcer on the calf. It began six months earlier and spread, discharging purulent material which grew no specific organism. Multiple antibiotic courses were impotent. On questioning, the captain described a six-month episode of bloody diarrhoea ten years earlier, and colonoscopy revealed burnt-out colitis with stricture formation. Six weeks of prednisolone therapy resulted in healing, leaving a papery scar (**818**).

Impressed by the destructive necrotic and non-infective ulceration of the skin, the Greek captain's interpreter said: 'Look—it is pyoderma'—using *pyoderma* as a Greek descriptive term! In such cases, it can be profitable to listen to the inter-preter as well as the patient. The condition may appear in association with inflammatory bowel disease (Crohn's disease and ulcerative colitis), collagen disease such as rheumatoid arthritis, and systemic lupus erythematosus—as well as reticulo-endothelial conditions.

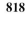

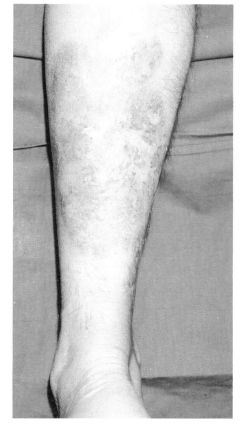

Viral infections

Human wart viruses belong to the genera papilloma-virus, a part of the papovavirus group of DNA viruses. Most are oncogenic. Human papilloma-viruses 1 and 2 (HPV 1, HPV 2) are the most frequent cause of plantar and palmar warts; HPV 4 causes punctata-like plantar warts, and HPV 7 is associated with papillomatous lesions.

819

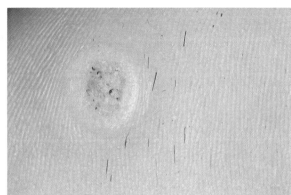

82

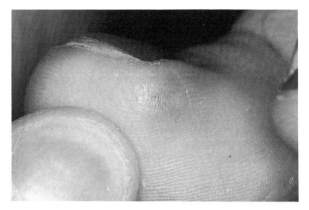

821

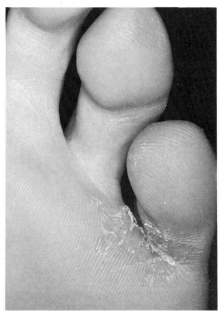

819 Plantar wart. The plantar wart is seen as a small shining grain-like papule with a rough kera-totic surface surrounded by a smooth collar of thickened horn. The epidermal ridges are not continued over the surface of the wart. There is a discrete area of hyperkeratosis where the epidermal ridges are not continued over the surface. On weight-bearing areas the proliferating tissue is pushed into the subcutaneous tissue causing pain. Small punctate dark areas are thrombosed capillaries in the dermal papillae.

820–822 Verruca pedis. This wart, adjacent to the nail fold, has had its thickened surface pared away with a scalpel, revealing the small bleeding points of the tips of elongated dermal papillae. Interdigital warts (**821 and 822**) may crack and be painful. The dermal papillae show as dots.

822

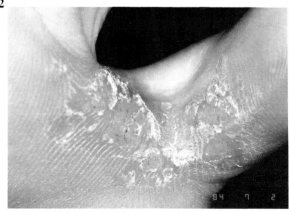

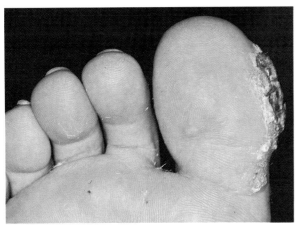

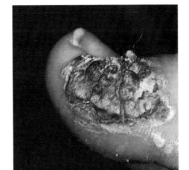
824

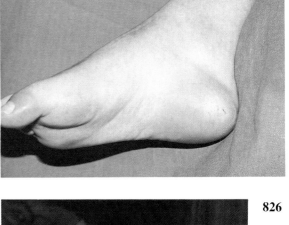
825

823 and 824 Plantar wart. A thick horny surface over the side of a great toe wart is surrounded by small satellite warts on the plantar surface of the toe and on the sole at the base of the 3rd toe under the metatarsal head.

825 Plantar wart *versus* pressure callus. The wart is often sited beneath a pressure point (in **823**, it is at the side of the toe). This thickened callosity of the heel complicates spina bifida and is caused by the abnormal weight distribution. This site is common to both wart and callus, but there are no dermal papillae to see. The plantar wart can be differentiated from a simple callosity by the fact that the epidermal ridges are interrupted over the wart and the ridges continue over the callus. The foot rolls inwards with each step and the skin creases that are produced can be seen above the callus. The skin over the 1st metatarsal head has a non weight-bearing appearance as the body weight pivots around the heel. A surgical scar of a tendon transplant overlays the dorsum.

826 A kidney transplant and warts. Immuno-suppression may account for the extensive plantar warts.

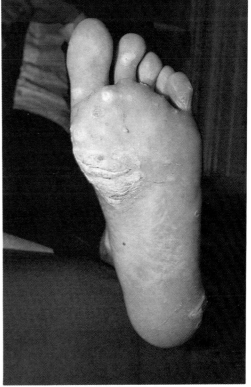
826

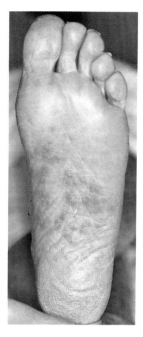
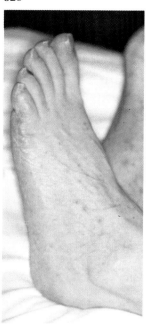

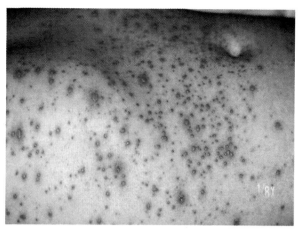

827–829 Chickenpox. The rash of varicella, a DNA herpes virus, may be seen in the feet as part of the generalised eruption of chickenpox. It is present as macules, papules and vesicles (polymorphic), and tends to be denser on the trunk (**829**). This man developed severe chickenpox post-operatively after a hernia operation; the initial fever led to some confusion until the typical rash appeared.

Fungal infections

In man, fungi can act as sensitisers or can invade tissues directly. When the immune system is depressed by drugs or the human immunodeficiency virus, fungi may produce life-threatening illness. More commonly, the infection is superficial—but nevertheless of importance, some 15 million people worldwide having been estimated to have ringworm of the scalp.[1]

Ringworm is produced by the effect of dermatophytes on the skin. The three genera responsible are *Microsporum*, *Trichophyton* and *Epidermophyton*. *Microsporum* may produce ringworm of the scalp in school children—*M. audovnii* and

M. canis are common (they fluoresce green under Wood's light). The dermatophytes are keratophilic and do not survive in serum. In keratin, they are protected from some serum-inhibitory property. *T. rubrum* rarely invades hair yet often invades nail; *E. flocculosum* does not invade hair and invades nail only occasionally.

The effect of ringworm on the skin depends on the extent of the inflammatory response which it engenders—ranging from *T. rubrum*'s quiet effect on the palms to the reactive kerion of *T. verrucosum* infections. Ringworm may mimic many skin diseases and become secondarily infected.

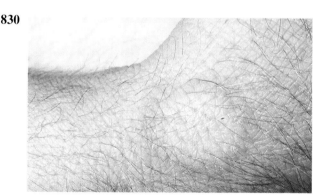

830 Tinea corporis—classic ringworm. The characteristic annular ringworm may reflect immunological changes. Growth continues at the edge but fungal mycelium is eliminated centrally and shows little propensity to regrow, opting preferentially for the edge.

Antigens diffusing from hyphae in the stratum corneum are presented to the immune system by epidermal Langerhan's cells. Cellular immunity is of great importance in the host's defence against ringworm, and accounts for the high incidence of fungal infections in AIDS.

[1]Grin, E. L. *Mycopathol. Mycol. Appl.*, 1964, **24**: 243.

In *Trichophyton rubrum* infections the inflammatory response appears simultaneously with the first demonstration, by skin testing, of delayed hypersensitivity. Regression of fungus infection may occur because cellular antibodies, by producing an inflammatory reaction in the dermis, allow the permeation of a serum inhibitory factor which kills the fungus.[2] Sensitised lymphocytes may play a part directly. Chronicity may correlate with atopy and acquired T-cell deficiency may account for the incidence in lymphoma and AIDS. The exuberance of the infection, if it is treated with topical steroids, may also be related to T-cell changes.

831 Ringworm in skin folds. Dry dermis is more resistant to infection, which may account for ringworm's predilection for sweaty toe clefts and skin folds. The active red scaly edge contrasts with the inactive central zone. The clinical picture results from a combination of the effects of keratin destruction and the host inflammatory response.[3] Some species have a predilection for a particular part of the body—*Microsporum audouinii*, tinea capitis, *Trichophyton rubrum*, tinea pedis (yet both may cause tinea corporis).

832–834 Tinea pedis (foot ringworm, athlete's foot). A foot infection with a dermatophyte fungus, usually *Trichophyton rubrum*, *T. interdigitale* or *Epidermophyton floccosum*. Suspect clinically and confirm by direct microscopy and culture. The macerated toe cleft skin predisposes to infection initially in a web space of the lateral toe clefts; lack of maceration may explain the rarity in those who habitually go barefoot. The sole, toe cleft or nails may be affected. Peeling, maceration and fissuring affects the toe cleft, and may spread to involve the sole (**832**) with peeling, scaling or vesiculobullous formation—particularly with *T. interdigitale*. Fissuring and peeling are seen in the interdigital cleft of this woman aged 60 (**833**), and on the 2nd and 3rd toes of this 25-year-old man—both wear shoes (**834**).

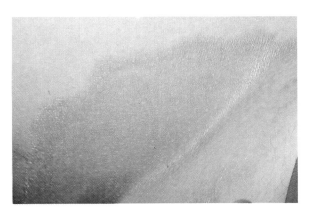

831

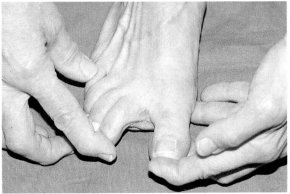

832

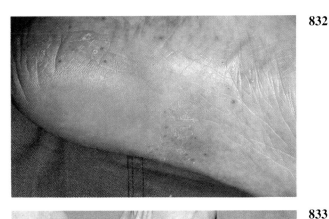

833

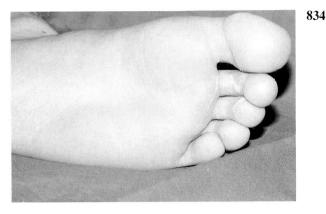

834

[2]Ahmed, A. R. 'Immunology of human dermatophyte infections.' *Arch. Dermatol.* 1982, **118**: 521.

[3]Further reading: Rook, *et al. Textbook of Dermatology* (5th ed, 1992).

835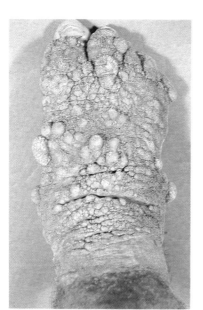

835 Chromoblastomycosis (verrucous dermatitis). A chronic fungal infection of the skin with a multiple aetiology, usually *Phialophora verrucosa* and *P. pedrosoi*. These fungi are found in the soil in rural communities. This Yoruba farmer in western Nigeria was uncomplaining of his very chronic problem.

836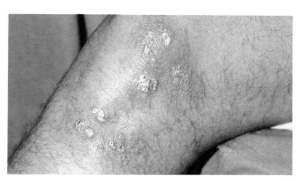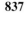

Parasitic infections

836 and 837 Cutaneous leishmaniasis (Delhi boil, Oriental sore). Due to infection with a protozoan, *Leishmania tropica*, *aethiopica* and *major*—Old World parasites; and *L. mexicana* and *brasiliensis*—new world parasites. It is transmitted by the bite of sandflies and is prevalent on the borders of the Mediterranean, Arabia, and central America.

This Riyadh resident spent a weekend in a rural oasis and sustained sandfly bites to the legs. Three weeks later he developed a red furuncle-like nodule which ulcerated and was associated with several satellite nodules in adjacent lymphatics. This rural zoonosis ulcerates, and heals leaving a scar.[4]

837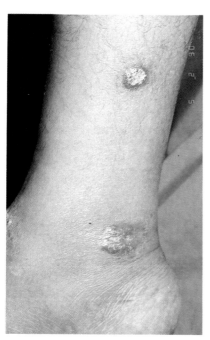

[4]Clinico-path. conference for discussion and differential diagnosis. Cutaneous Leishmaniasis. *N. Eng. J. M.* Feb. 14, 1991.

838 Guinea worm. Infestation with the adult female *Dracunculus medinensis*, which ends her life cycle here. The white worm is protruding through a broken blister and is being wound onto a stick. A second blister adjacent to the worm is caused by a second female. The nematode, which is widely distributed in Africa and Asia, discharges large numbers of ova on contact with water, and the larvae must be ingested by cyclops water fleas. Inadvertent human consumption of water containing the flea leads to the liberation, within the body, of the larvae, which then migrate into loose retroperitoneal tissue where they take up to 12 months to mature into the adult worm. The gravid female then migrates downwards and ultimately a blister is formed which bursts on contact with water and the worm discharges its ova. Worms frequently become lost, then calcify; they may be palpated beneath the skin or seen on X-ray. The main complication is sepsis.

839 and 840 Scabies of the wrist and finger. Pruritus is the cardinal symptom of infestation with the mite of human scabies, *Sarcoptes scabiei*. The diagnosis is made on the distribution of the lesions and the finding of the characteristic burrows and mite. However, the secondary changes from itching may blur the picture, and the 15-year cycle of epidemics may lead to medical unfamiliarity. Irregular crusting, thickening and fissuring of the skin of the soles and hands may be misdiagnosed in a very extensive infestation (Norwegian scabies, described by the Norwegian, Cesar Boeck).

The 0.2×0.15 mm female mite lays her eggs in burrows and then dies; the eggs hatch and the larvae emerge in three to four days before making their way to the skin surface. Favoured sites help in diagnosis. In 85% of human males mites are carried on the hands and wrists; in 30–40% on the elbows, feet, ankles and genitals. In the human female the palms and the nipples are favoured. Infestation on the head is rare—pilosebaceous-bearing skin is shunned. A typical load is 50 oviparous female mites, and spread is by close physical contact (often sexual). An allergic hypersensitivity to the mite products leads to pruritus with a rise in IgG and IgM; the itch is worse at night. The burrows can be seen on the anterior aspect of the wrist and between the finger webs (see **839** and **840**). A vesicle is seen on the thumb; it is usually at the end of a burrow. Secondary infection occurs.

838

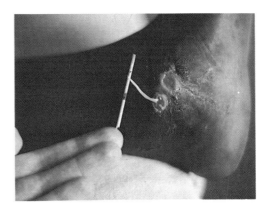

839

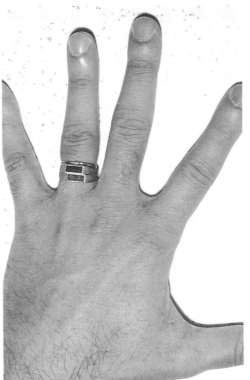

840

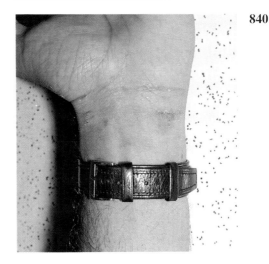

Sensitisation and irritation

Irritation may result from something as prosaic as water which is hypotonic and which may—in the right climate—dissolve the hygroscopic substances which keep the skin supple. Skin-cleaning agents used at work may do more damage than the dirt itself! Perhaps the feet are lucky, in that they are less exposed and less washed, although their coverings and treatment may lead to irritation or sensitisation.

Sensitisation with a substance leads to allergic contact dermatitis mediated by cellular immunity — conjugation of the substance with a protein leads to hapten formation. This antigen complex leads to the production of sensitised lymphocytes. Subsequent contact with the allergen elicits a T-cell lymphocyte response with the appearance of eczema at the site.

Up to 30 per cent of allergic contact dermatitis may be related to sensitivity to medicaments or their vehicles, particularly in the case of substances applied to stasis eczema and ulcers on the legs, especially if an occlusive dressing is used.

841

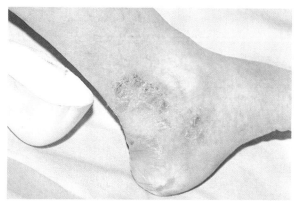

841 Irritation by proprietary polyethylene foam? The scars of an old pressure sore on the apex of the heel and the lesion from shoe rub at the Achilles' tendon insertion have been protected by a polyethylene foam pad—sensitivity to these plastics is very uncommon. Irritation at the edge of the heel cup has produced skin damage from friction, and maceration around the scar (the pad had been worn next to the skin). Hypostatic eczema and fungal infections must be excluded but once the relationship of the skin change to the contact area of the foam is noted then the cause is clear.

842

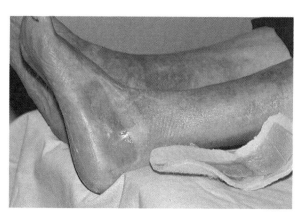

843

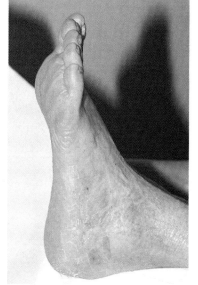

842 and 843 The effect of occlusion on scarred skin. An attempt had been made to protect the extensive thin scar on the lateral foot by applying a foam pad. The insertion of a hydrocolloid gel in a polyisobutylene adhesive mass between the scarred skin and the foam pad has led to this reaction in the abnormal skin. Once air circulates (**843**) the reaction subsides.

844 Shoe dermatitis. The rash usually spares the interdigital clefts. It may be due to rubber, chromates or dyes used in the shoe manufacture. The pattern of sensitisation will depend on whether the agent is present in the upper or the sole of the shoe. The pattern here is typical of Arabian or Indian sandals which have a strap between the first and second clefts and across the dorsum of the instep, corresponding to the contact area with the leather. Sensitisation is caused by the chrome sulphate used in tanning of the leather of these Middle-Eastern sandals. Chromate is rarely used in Europe and North America but formaldehyde resin may be incorporated into cheap foot wear and produce a similar problem.

This man knew he was sensitised but loved his sandals too much. If he has many pairs then at least the sweat has less chance to leach the chemical out if he changes them regularly!

Chrome metal forms an oxide on the surface which is relatively inert and sensitises infrequently, by contrast with nickel.

845 and 846 Nickel contact dermatitis. A very common sensitiser more frequently seen in women than men: usually present as a plating or as an alloy in jewellery[5] or fasteners in clothing. It is ubiquitous—small amounts may be found even in detergents. Since contact dermatitis can mimic most eruptions, diagnosis requires suspicion and a careful history. The distribution is a valuable clue, as in this eczematous necklace rash echoed in the ear lobe and adjacent to the wrist watch strap buckle (**846**). Contrast this with the rash in flexural scabies which is not so localised (**840**). Sometimes the contact may be less clear but analysis leads to diagnosis.

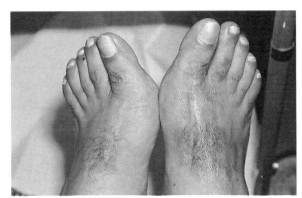

844

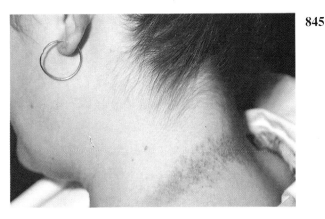

845

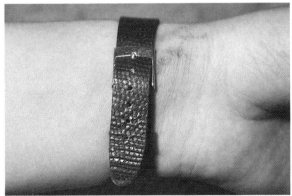
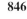

846

[5]Compare this with the scabies itch which *is not* under the watch strap and its buckle (**840**).

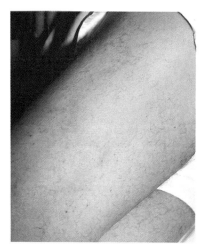 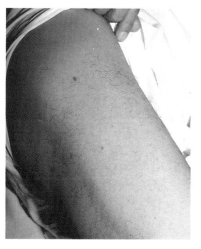 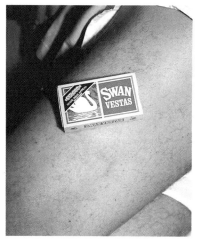

847–849 Phosphorus sesquisulphide sensitivity. A patch of eczema on the thigh (left thigh, **847**), but if simple eczema it should be bilateral and often symmetrical (right thigh, **848** clear)—so a contact relationship is a possibility. This skin is overlain by the trouser pocket where a right-handed smoker keeps his red-tipped strike-anywhere matches. The phosphorus sesquisulphide leaches through the cloth to the skin.

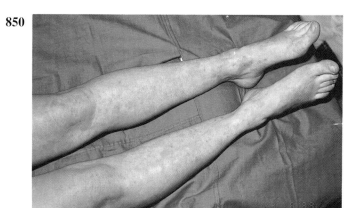 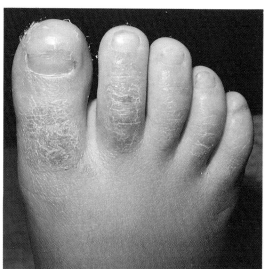

850 and 851 Atopy of the legs and foot. The skin is often affected symmetrically and this usually involves the limb flexures, neck and ankles. The extensor aspects may also be involved. On the dorsum of the toes true eczematous lesions may occur; these are often discoid in shape.

Miscellaneous vasculitic phenomena

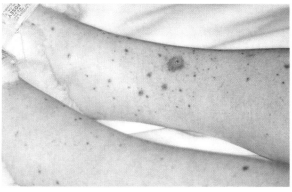

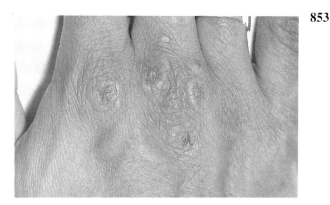

852–856 Erythema multiforme. A distinctive clinical and histological entity which may be precipitated by a variety of stimuli: infection with viruses such as herpes simplex, streptococci, tuberculosis, mycoplasma; connective tissue disease—SLE; or drugs—sulphonamides and topical applications. It may recur and vary greatly in severity and form. The mechanism is immunological and may be associated with immune complex formation, which when severe may affect the mouth, eyes, skin (**854, 855**) and genitalia—**the Stevens–Johnson syndrome.**[6] The mucous membranes may develop a characteristic membrane (**856**). Systemic upset may be severe. It may recur. The simple lesion is a dull red maculo-papule whose centre may become purpuric and look like a target or iris (**853**). A central bulla may be present.

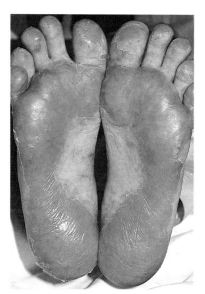

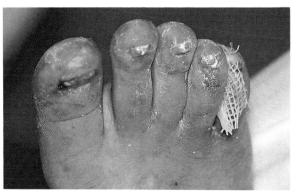

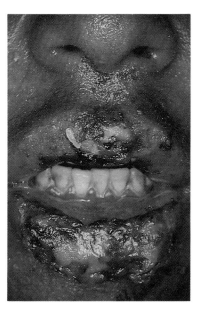

[6]**Albert Mason Stevens,** American physician 1884–1945, **Frank Craig Johnson,** American paediatrician 1894–1934, described in 1922.

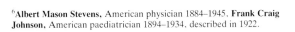

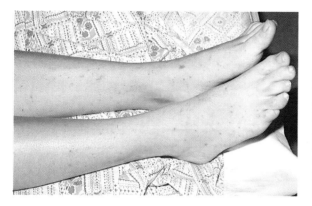

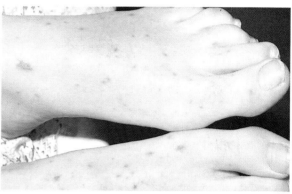

857 and 858 Anaphylactoid or Henoch–Schönlein[7] purpura. Non-thrombocytopaenia purpura with urticarial onset, related to immune complex formation in response to a variety of stimuli, often streptococcal. Children predominate. Oedema, joint pains of the knees and ankles and abdominal pains are often seen. Microscopic haematuria reflects renal involvement.

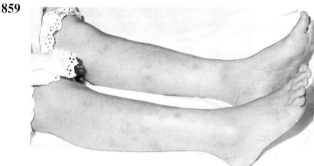

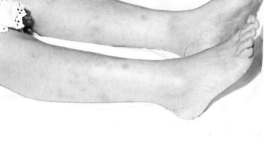

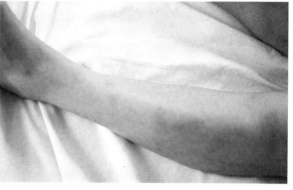

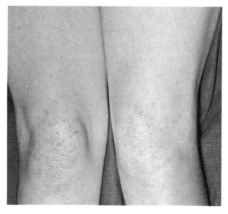

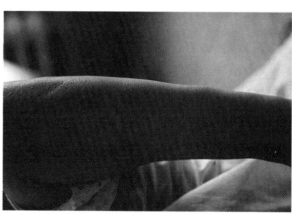

859–862 Erythema nodosum. These nodular lumps on the shins or extensor aspects of the arms (**862**) may be tender and red. The colour changes like a bruise. The onset is abrupt and may be associated with fever and arthralgia. It may recur and usually subsides over 3 to 6 weeks. Its recognition should prompt thought about the underlying cause. This is a hypersensitivity vasculitis in response to a variety of stimuli which include infections (streptococcal, mycoplasma, tuberculosis) or in association with sarcoidosis, ulcerative colitis or drugs such as sulphonamides.

[7]**Eduard Heinrich Henoch,** German physician 1820–1910 described 1868. **Johann Lukas Schönlein,** German physician 1792–1864 described 1832.

Psoriasis

A common, genetically determined chronic skin disease with sharply demarcated red plaques, seen particularly on certain sites—knees, elbows, scalp, sacrum and penis. There is enormous morphological variation. Nail changes occur. It may be complicated by joint disease.

863

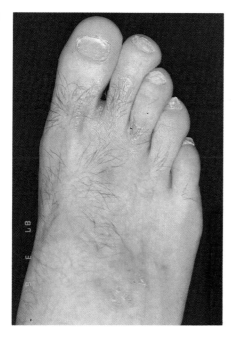

864

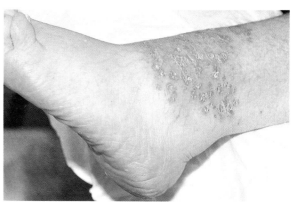

865

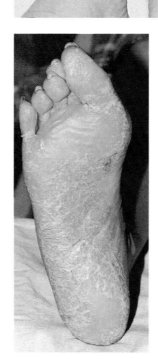

863 The lifting of the nail plate (onycholysis) and shedding of the nail may be caused by trauma, fungal infection, skin disease like lichen planus and alopecia areata, or be part of the nail changes seen in psoriasis; the red nummular plaques with a silvery scale can be seen on the toes.

864 and 865 Guttate psoriatic lesions varying in size from 0.5 to 1.0cm in diameter on the lower part of the leg with the silver scale. The nail may be grossly thickened or shed (**865**). A plaque is present on the left foot.

866 Psoriasis of the sole. On the sole, psoriasis is present as scaly patches where the fine silver scale can be produced by scratching.

866

867   **868**   **869**

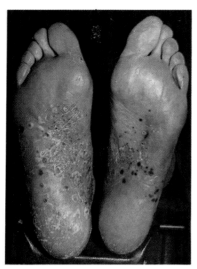 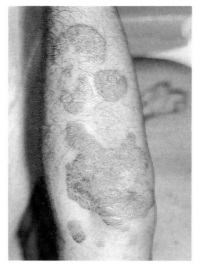 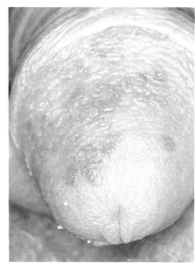

867 Pustular psoriasis. A pustulosis may occur sometimes in association with rupioid lesions — limpet-like lesions with hyperkeratosis.

868 Psoriatic plaque on elbow. Psoriasis may occur at sites of trauma or scars and exhibits the Koebner phenomenon[8] in which disease appears in previously traumatised skin as well as being present elsewhere. It may be seen in psoriasis, in lichen planus, active eczema and molluscum contagiosum. If the lesions are sparse then other sites should be examined.

869 Psoriasis of the glans penis. Psoriasis may be present on the skin of the uncircumcised penis, where it will lack scales.

870

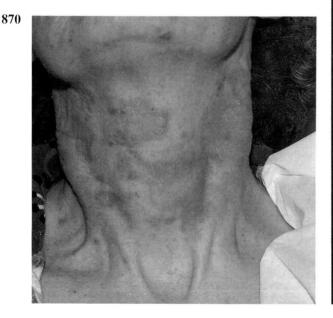

871

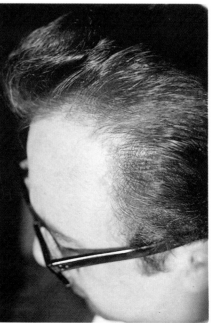

870 The neck. The red plaques have silvery scales.

[8]**Heinrich Koebner,** German dermatologist 1838–1904. (1877) *Viert fur Dermatol Syphil 8,559.*

871 The scalp. Very thick plaques may occur, though the hair itself may be unaffected. All the scalp may be affected or only discrete patches found.

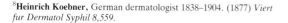

Tumours

The possibility of a malignant lesion of the foot should always be considered in the differential diagnosis. Basal cell carcinoma may occur on the sole of the foot and subungual melanoma be mistaken for a linear naevus of the nail or a haematoma. Spontaneous thrombosis in a plantar wart becomes clear if the surface is pared down.

872

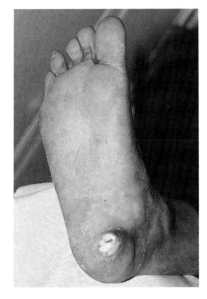

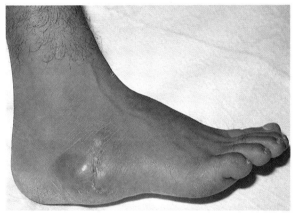
873

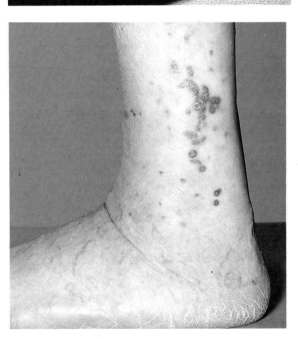
874

875

872 Squamous cell carcinoma. A malignant tumour which variably metastasises, it occurs rarely on the sole. An Asian man with poor English, no interpreter plus difficulty in history taking led to incorrect early treatment; it had been mistaken for a wart.

873 Melanoma. A melanoma may occur at any site. It may not be pigmented. On the foot subungual and plantar ones may occur and a high index of suspicion is essential. A pigmented lesion on the foot which the patient thinks is changing in any way should be removed and examined histologically.

874–877 Kaposi's sarcoma (HIV negative).[9] A male of 83 with an indolent red plaque (**874**). It often affects the distal extremities and is more common in older persons in contrast to its distribution in those infected with the human immunodeficiency virus (HIV), when any part of the body may be affected, and there is no specific age band. It occurs throughout Europe and is not restricted to specific ethnic groups. It is particularly common in Africa. Bluish red or dark brown nodules or plaques may appear black on a dark skin and lead to diagnostic confusion. The plaques may fuse and oedema of limb develop.

[9]**Moritz Kaposi–Kohn,** Hungarian dermatologist 1837–1902. 'Lichen ruber moniliformis.' *Vjschr. Derm.*, 1886, **13:** 571.

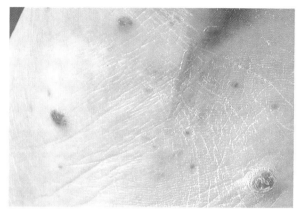

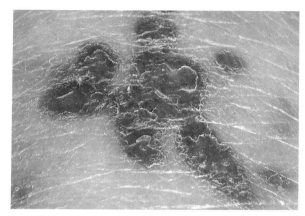

The rate of growth is variable but may be rapid in Africans (**884**). In this leg the plaques have fused but if a single lesion is examined then the typical flat-topped plaque is seen just like the bluish red one on a pale skin (**881**).

878

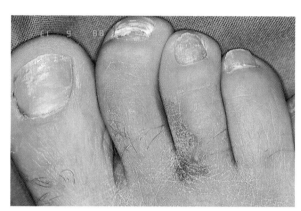

879

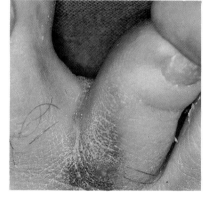

878 and 879 HIV-positive Kaposi's sarcoma with onycholysis and folliculitis. This young man complained of intractable shedding of the toe nails over a six-month period: there was onycholysis and, since he was a dancer, trauma was felt likely to be a factor. No skin lesions to suggest a general cause such as psoriasis were found on general examination. Culture of the nail showed the cause to be fungal infection, but treatment was ineffective. He complained that his skin was dry and flaky—unusual in a normal youth whose skin was usually moist and sweaty. An inflamed hair follicle with pus was noted on the third toe and another on the fourth. These two infections in a young male suggested impaired immune response. The urine was free from sugar. Overlying the second interdigital cleft there was a purple plaque whose significance became clear (**879**)—Kaposi's sarcoma in a homosexual male who is HIV positive.

—dry skin
—fungal infection → red plaque = ? AIDS.
—folliculitis

Kaposi's sarcoma occurs in:
- elderly males-*sporadic*-unassociated with HIV
- in subsaharan Africa-*endemic*-before HIV
- in AIDS-*epidemic*-especially in homosexuals
- *iatrogenic*-immunosuppression in renal transplants

880

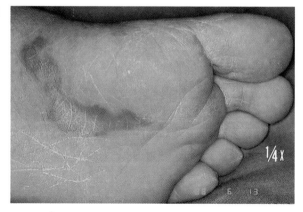

880 HIV-positive Kaposi on the sole of the foot.

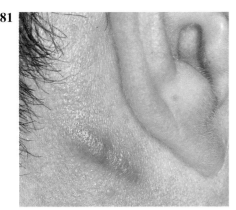

881

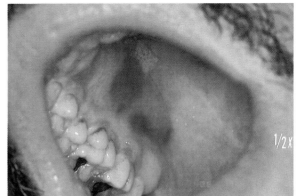

882

881 A typical plaque of Kaposi's sarcoma.

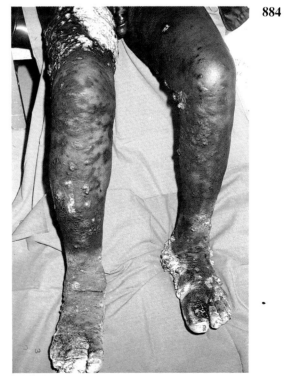

883

882 and 883 HIV. Kaposi's sarcoma on the palate, and oral candidiasis. It is easy to miss lesions on the hard palate unless one specifically looks, for the glance down the throat misses the palate. Kaposi's sarcoma may be asymptomatic. A plaque of monilia is present which is not found in the normal individual. Oral candidiasis may be present in 50 per cent of AIDS patients[10] and may be the first sign of infection, seen on the soft palate (**883**).

884 Kaposi's sarcoma, African feet. Extensive plaques are present, which coalesce in places. If an individual plaque is analysed then the diagnosis is easier. The white areas are calamine lotion—often applied by patients to their skin and leading to diagnostic confusion in the novice.

885 Tattoo in drug addict. Do not forget that other clues to the risk factors of HIV infection may be easily seen if looked for—this man presented with septicaemia and had track marks from repeated intravenous injection on his arms. These may be immediately apparent, though less obvious sites are often used. The chest X-ray (above) shows a lung abscess with a visible fluid level.

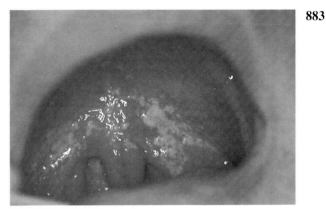

884

885

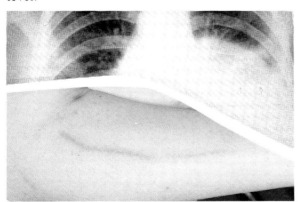

[10]Cook, G. C. 'The mouth in HIV infection.' *Quart. J. Med.*, July 1990.

Miscellaneous conditions affecting the skin

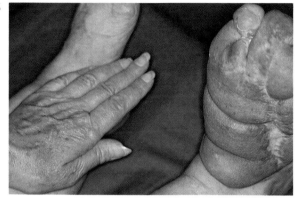

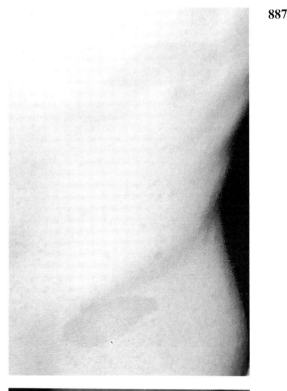

886 Neurofibromatosis (NF type I[11]). This condition is transmitted as an autosomal dominant disease, with high penetrance but varying expression. It usually occurs as a new mutation. (It is seen even in fishes.) The defect on chromosome 17 produces a clinical picture of *café-au-lait* spots, cutaneous neurofibromata and other associated defects, many involving neural crest-derived tissues. In the lower limb, plexiform neuromas may occur and envelop the part, as here, and pseudoarthroses of the tibia may occur. Type II NF is due to a defect on chromosome 22. It may have sparse cutaneous manifestations but can be associated with bilateral acoustic neuromata and no iris hamartomata.[12]

887 *Café-au-lait* spots. The *café-au-lait* spots may appear in childhood and be accompanied by the development of a variable number of cutaneous neurofibromata (**889 and 890**).

888 Plexiform neuromas. The plexiform neuroma develops from cutaneous plexi and may envelop the digit or limb. It is a characteristic change in NF.

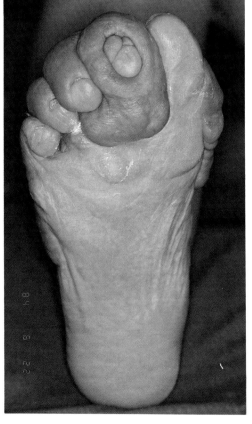

[11]Described by *Frederick Daniel von Recklinghausen*, German pathologist, 1833–1910. His patient had *café-au-lait* spots and neuromata as well as gastrointestinal lesions. The presence of plexiform lesions is characteristic. Iris hamartomata occur in all affected patients by the age of 21. If *café-au-lait* spots, neuromata and iris nodules are absent by the teens, the chance of inheritance is negligible.

A very full description of this fascinating disease is given in two articles: 'Clin. Path. Conf.' *N. Eng. J. Med.*, 1989, **320**: 996. 'Lisch nodules in NF Type I.' *N. Eng. J. Med.*, 1991, **324**: 1264.

[12]Martuza and Eldrige. 'Neurofibromatosis Type 2.' *N. Eng. J. Med.*, 1988, **318**: 684.

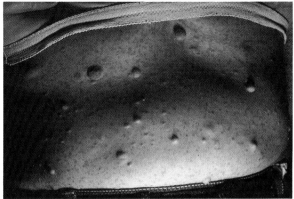

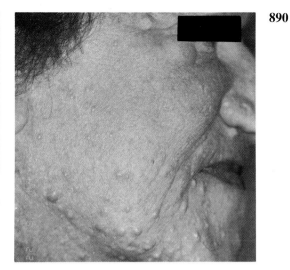

889 and 890 Cutaneous neurofibromata on the abdomen and face.

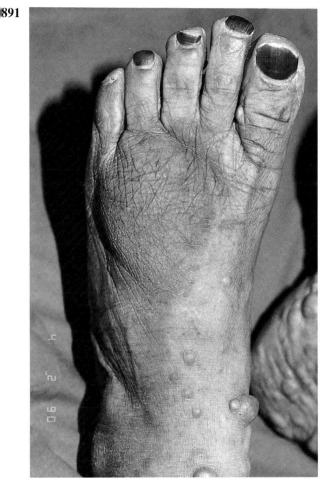

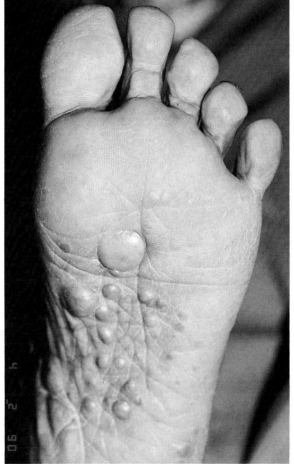

891 and 892 Plexiform neuroma (Type I NF). This foot has a dorsal plexiform neuroma overlain by a *café-au-lait* spot. There are numerous small cutaneous neuromata over the dorsum of the foot, and on the sole (**892**) they occur over the non weight-bearing area.

893

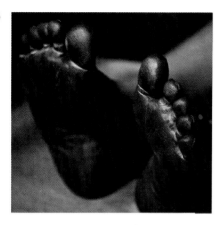

894

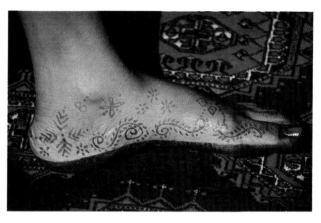

893 and 894 Henna[13] and the feet. Henna is a vegetable dye also used to colour the hair, and to decorate the skin. Patterns may be formed of great intricacy on the feet and hands (**894**), colouring the nails. It may be used in the belief that it will toughen the skin of the feet of Arabian gulf pearl divers, to colour the hair of the elderly, or be applied to the head as a relief for headache. It may be used on the nails where it stains rather than coats the nail. To the devout Moslem who wishes to wash before prayer it is preferable to nail varnish: henna produces a colouring coat 'per-meable' to water and permits cleansing before prayer. The time elapsed since it was applied can be gauged by the amount that the nail has grown out and is undyed. On the palms, which may be stained when the hair has been coloured, there is a trap for the unwary to see pigmented palmar creases and invoke an elevated ACTH level as the reason (see **509**). Modern dyes such as para-phenylenediamine may be mixed with henna to speed up the dyeing process and lead to sensitisation. Henna doesn't sensitise.

895
896

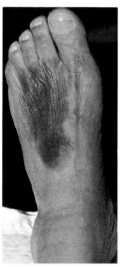

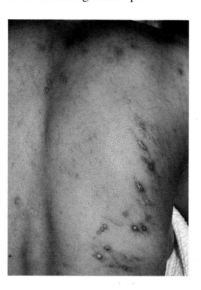

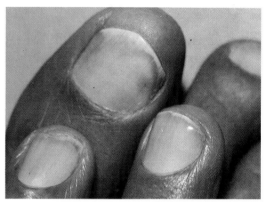

89·

895 Lichen aureus. A golden brown plaque which has a lichenoid histology and may be localised anywhere—first described on the eyelid—needs no treatment and is rare.

896 and 897 Scratch marks and the skin. Lichenification and pigmentation may be the result of friction due to scratching. These marks are confined to the area of the back that the patient can reach. The question that must be answered is 'WHY does this person scratch?'. Then the diagnosis will not be missed and may range from senile pruritus to infestations and include malignancy, cholestasis, diabetes mellitus and neurodermatitis. The chronic pruritic will have buffed finger-nail tips like mirrors yet the toe-nails will be matte (**897**).

[13]The oriental shrub al-henna (arabic)—the Egyptian privet. Its leaves and young shoots. 1646: Sir Thomas Browne—'Alcanna being greene, will suddenly infect the nailes and other parts with a durable red.' *Pseud. Epid.* 383.

242

898 Ainhum and its differential diagnosis. A constricting band is present around the fifth toe and may deepen and lead to auto-amputation. Pseudo-ainhum may occur secondary to another condition. Ainhum is a common condition in Africa, and this Nigerian farmer's only complaint was of pain if the foot was knocked. The differential diagnosis includes trauma in lepers and other neuropathies, progressive systemic sclerosis and rare palmo-plantar keratoderma and other hereditary diseases.

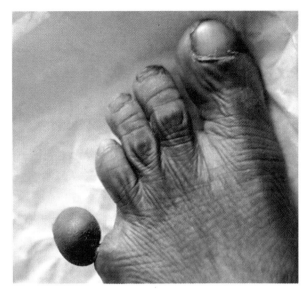

The nails[14]
Neglect

The potential medical significance of the neglected foot must be appreciated. Causes include senility, mental and physical disability, alcohol and drug addiction, hypothyroid states, diabetes with the wilful neglect syndrome or diabetic retinopathy and those blind from other causes.

Seeing a neglected foot must trigger the query . . . WHY?

899 Neglected feet. These feet have to belong to an individual with an important socio-medical problem. Unless that is appreciated, the chance to help may be missed. A 42-year-old male schizophrenic who lives in the community, his hygiene is poor: though the feet have been superficially washed the ingrained dirt persists. He neglects to cut the nails.

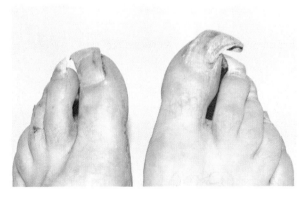

899

---

[14]Onychomancy—Divination from the finger nails—1855 Smedley. *Occult Sci.* 324. Chiromancers give the name of Onycomancy, likewise, to the inspection of the natural signs in the nails (*OED*).

Traumatic disorders of the nail

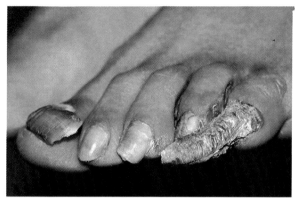

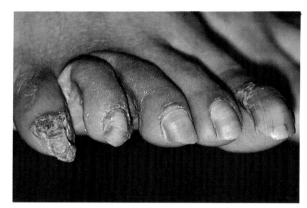

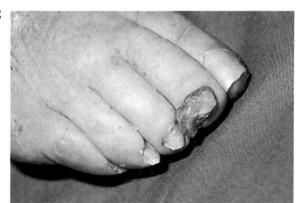

900–902 Onychogryphosis.[15] A thickened nail is difficult to cut and so is allowed to grow, becoming moulded by the shoe. Trauma may be the initiating factor and accounts for the term 'ostler's nail', (the ostler's feet were trodden on when he was tending horses at a hostelry).[16] Note the stages (**900**) of thickening of the curved second toe-nail, the middle ridged from pressure and the first and fifth with the fully developed entity. The shape (**902**) of the second toe-nail may account for the description 'ram's horn nail'.

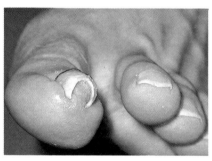

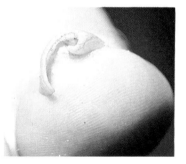

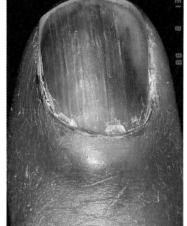

903 and 904 Involuted great toe-nail. The nail is rolled in at the edges; it may be congenital or precipitated by the lateral squeeze produced by footwear. Here the tendency for the other nails to involute can be seen in the second and third toes. A futile attempt has been made (**903**) to correct this with a nail brace.

905 Subungual haematoma. Crushing leads to subungual bleeding which, if unevacuated, may lead to loss of the nail.

[15]Onychogryphosis—Gr. Onychos, nail + *Gryphos*, hooking.
[16]Phonetic spelling of the historical hosteler with the h mute (Old French). The hosteler ran a hostelry and dealt with horses.

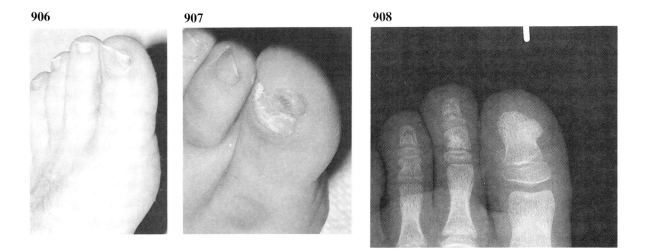

906–908 Subungual exostosis. This usually presents with pain due to outgrowth of bone on the terminal phalanx of the great toe, which lifts the nail. Removal leads to pain relief. The exostosis in **906**, seen on X-ray in **908**, must be dealt with.

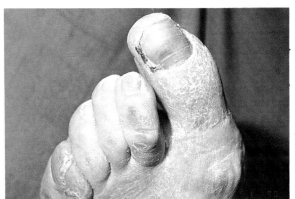

909 Shoe pressure in a diabetic. A one-hour flight wearing a new pair of tight shoes led to subsequent nail shedding in this insulin-dependent diabetic. Trauma led to onycholysis.

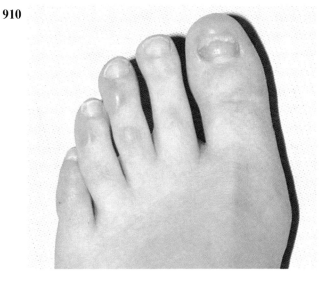

910 and 911 Acute onycholysis. A girl aged 20 with damage to the left great toe and the third and fourth toes from acute shoe rub. The toe-nail was shed but she persisted in skiing in borrowed ski boots which were too short. This led to permanent damage to the nail bed as the epidermis covered it. There is acute bursitis under the first metacarpophalangeal joint (**911**).

245

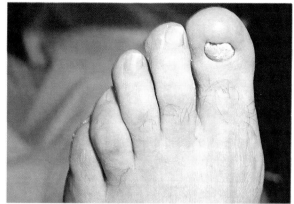

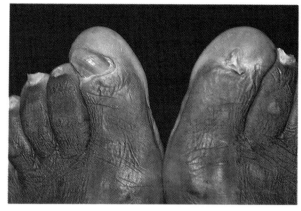

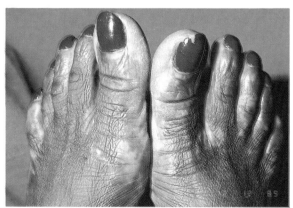

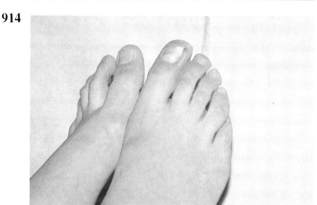

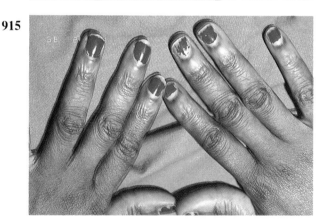

912 Onychogryphosis. The end result of old trauma to the nail bed and matrix is onychogryphosis (thickened and deformed nail plate) and onycholysis.

913 Chronic trauma. A Nigerian lawyer played football barefoot in his youth. This led to nail trauma and permanent damage. He preferred to kick right footed!

914 Onychocryptosis (penetration of nail sulcus by the nail). When a young person complains of an 'ingrowing' toe-nail they may refer to this; whereas an old person may refer to callus in the nail sulcus. The fourth and fifth toes are tucked under, and all toes show soft-tissue moulding suggesting footwear as the cause. Picking of the nail rather than cutting may contribute to the problem.

915 and 916 Lacquered nails. Nail polish will wear more on the hand most used—normally the dominant side—but nervously picking at the varnish may be done by the dominant hand and confuse the deductions! The date of the last application can be deduced from the distance that the nail has grown (rate of growth = 1–2 mm a week). Here the right-handed woman has picked the worn nail varnish with the left hand—the dominant hand has shorter finger nails. Toe-nails grow more slowly and don't get so chipped: vitiligo is present (**916**). Henna, when used to stain the nail, doesn't chip but does grow out (**894**).

Growth disorders of the nails

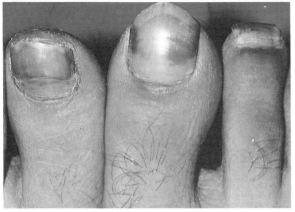

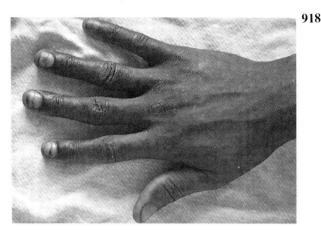

917 and 918 Growth arrest lines. Transverse lines on the nail may denote growth arrest and the lapse of time since the event can be gauged by the distance that the line has moved. Systemic illness or local ischaemia may be the reason. Here the lines are local, from unilateral ischaemia due to an embolus (**917**), and bilaterally from a systemic illness (smallpox) leading to the lines seen in the finger nails (**918**) and the scars on the dorsum of the hand. Fingernails grow at about 1 mm/wk and toe-nails more slowly—about 0.5 mm/wk. So the chronology is written on the finger!

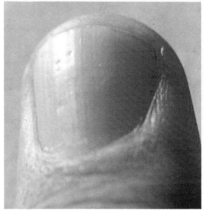

919

919 Pitting of the nail. Abnormal areas of keratin may be formed if the matrix is affected in psoriasis, eczema, fungus infection and chronic paronychia, alopecia areata, and sometimes in normal healthy people. These areas of parakeratosis may fall off leaving pits. The nail may grow faster than a normal nail.

920 Pitting of the nails. This woman with psoriasis has well-marked nail pitting and a swollen terminal interphalangeal joint with a seronegative polyarthritis.

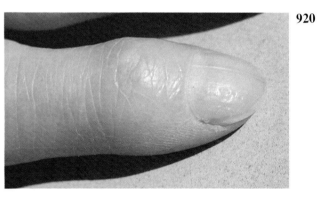

920

921 Onycholysis of the nails.[17] Separation of the nail from the nail bed. It is commonly related to trauma, but may occur in peripheral ischaemia, with some skin diseases and in infections. It may be related to the occupation.

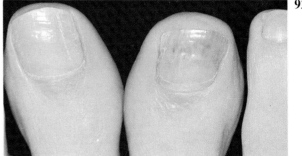

921

[17]Causes include trauma, fungal infection, psoriasis, lichen planus, thyroid disease and the yellow nail syndrome.

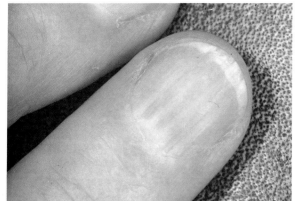

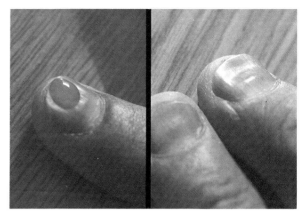

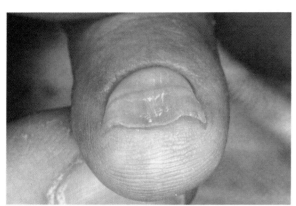

922 Ridging and beading of the nail. This may be a normal finding in an elderly person, but is also seen in lichen planus when all nails may be affected.

923A, B and 924 Koilonychia. The spoon-shaped nail is seen in young children. It may be part of a growth disorder of the nail in severe illness (**924**), as in this man with severe recurrent Stevens–Johnson syndrome; or, traditionally but rarely now, it is associated with iron-deficiency anaemia.

Clubbing of the nails

Clubbing of the nails describes the change produced by an increased amount of tissue, first seen at the base of the nail bed, which leads to sponginess and a change in the angle that the plate makes with the axis of the finger (**926**). As it progresses the end of the digit may assume a drumstick shape.

It is seen in association with chronic inflammatory lung disease, fibrosing lung disease, carcinoma of the bronchus, heart disease (bacterial endocarditis and cyanotic heart disease), chronic inflammatory bowel disease and in association with thyroid acropachy.

The trapping of particles of megakaryocytes with their platelet growth factor in the capillaries may lead to the vascular hyperplastic tissue and could explain the fact that the fingers are usually more grossly clubbed than the toes as the bits of megakaryocyte may be broken up before they arrive at the feet and don't get stuck.[18]

[18]Dickinson, C. J., Martin, J. F. 'Megakaryocytes and platelet clumps as the cause of finger clubbing.' *Lancet*, 1987, **ii:** 1434–35.

925

926

928

927

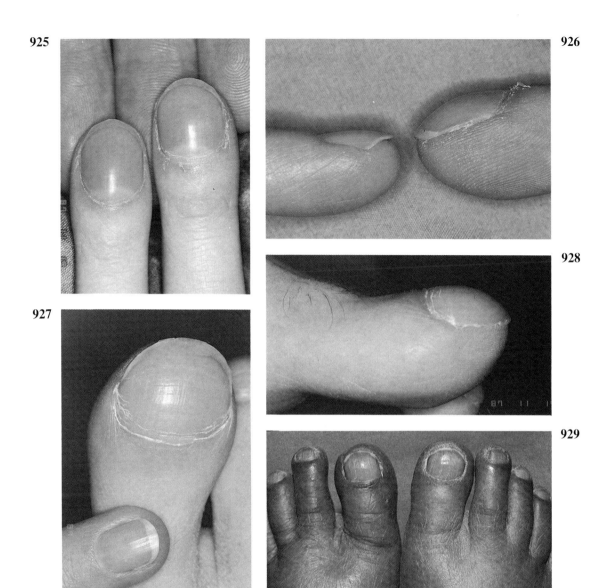

929

925–930 Nail clubbing. The first picture in this series shows young cyanosed clubbed fingers (**925**), so the differential diagnosis is tipped towards inflammatory lung disease—cystic fibrosis —rather than another disease which would affect an older person (**929**)—longstanding cryptogenic fibrosing alveolitis. The toes (**927, 930**) show transverse lines which may reflect acute episodes of lung infection—comparison with a normal finger helps to assess pallor and cyanosis.

930

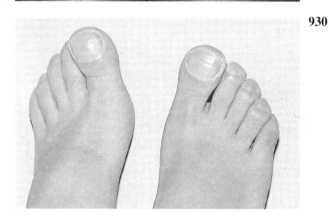

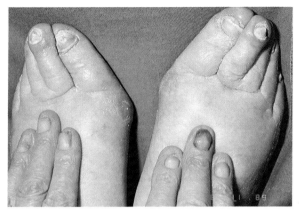

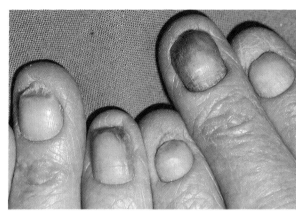

931 and 932 Yellow nail syndrome. This is a rare but characteristic condition. This lady had yellow/green, thick, slow-growing nails, onycholysis, peripheral oedema and bronchiectasis. First described by Samman and White (1964)[19] and associated with poor peripheral lymphatics, an association with pleural effusion and thickening and bronchiectasis occurs.[20]

Vascular disorders and the nail

The nail bed may reflect vasculitis as in rheumatoid arthritis and have infarcts in systemic sclerosis —as well as dilated capillary loops in other collagen diseases like lupus erythematosus and dermatomyositis.[21]

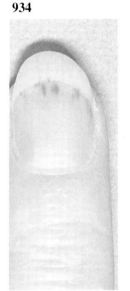

933–935 Splinters in the nail (splinter haemorrhages). Longitudinal haemorrhages, seen under the nail. This is a physical sign which, like so many, must be seen in perspective against the normal frequency of occurrence/epidemiology. It may occur in 26 to 56 per cent of normal people as a consequence of trauma; it is then seen more often in manual workers and in the dominant hand.[22] Splinters may be seen in bacterial endocarditis but are usually absent. Sometimes they are seen in individuals with indwelling arterial catheters. In this man (**933**) bacterial endocarditis (BE) on an aortic prosthetic valve is associated with splinter haemorrhages which may be embolic, from thrombus on the valve and a mycotic aneurysm of the popliteal artery (**935**).

[19]Samman and White. 'The yellow nail syndrome.' *Brit. J. Derm.,* **110:** 866.
[20]Emerson, Peter. 'Yellow nails, lymphoedema and pleural effusions.' *Thorax,* 1966, **21:**247.

[21]Samitz, M. H. 'Cuticular changes in dermatomyositis.' *Arch. Dermatol.,* 1974, **11:** 866.
[22]Young, J. B. *et al.* 'Splinter haemorrhages: fact and fiction.' *J. Roy. Coll. Phys. of London.,* **22:** 4, 240.

936 Emboli in BE. A combination of platelets and bacteria may lead to this condition.

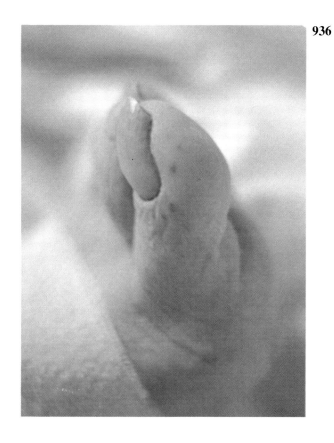

Dystrophic nails

937 Lichen planus in toe-nails. Nail changes occur in 10 per cent of cases and range from longitudinal ridging to loss of the nail. The cuticle may grow over the nail plate and attach to it, leading to pterygium unguis and permanent nail loss.

938 Lichen planus of fingernails. Pterygium formation has led to nail loss; beading can be seen in the little fingernail.

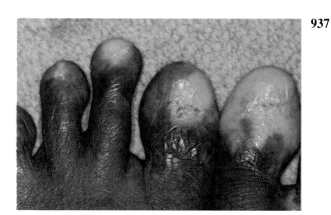

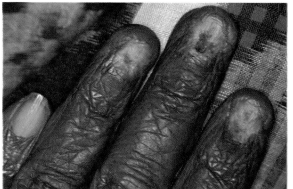

939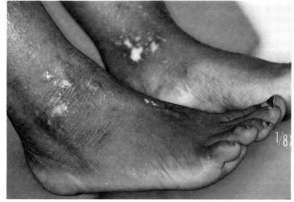

940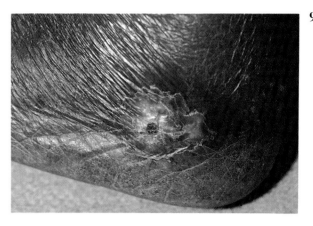

941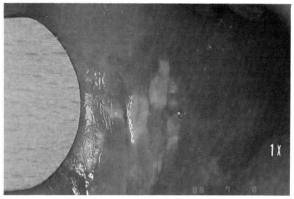

942

943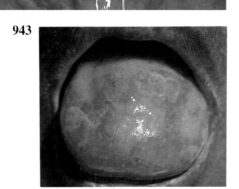

944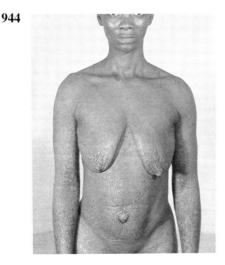

939–944 Lichen planus of the feet. Skin lesions in lichen planus are mauve, flat-topped, shiny papules over which may be seen a lace-like pattern. This may also be seen in the mouth (**941**). In the mouth a distinction must be made between lichen planus and leukoplakia, which is a premalignant disturbance of oral mucosal kera-tinisation. Leukoplakia (**942**) may be associated with candida, tobacco or trauma, while a variant hairy leukoplakia seen on the border of the tongue is associated with Epstein–Barr virus infection and AIDS. Glossitis may be a feature (**943**); note the absence of angular oral soreness. The rash may be seen on the flexor aspect of the wrist or around the ankle, but may be widespread (**944**) and affect any part of the body.

Infected nails

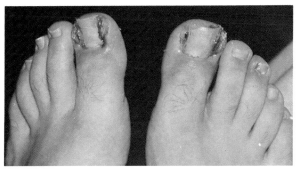

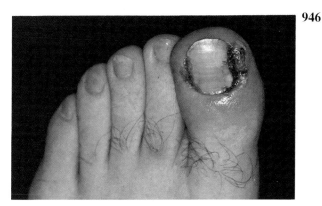

945–946 Paronychial infection of the toes. These two examples reflect the spectrum of infection related to onychocryptosis.

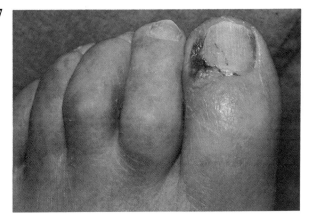

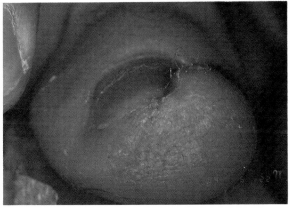

947 Ischaemia masquerading as sepsis. This was mistakenly treated as onychocryptosis by cutting the nail back.

948 Onychocryptosis. The side of the nail has been cut to relieve the discomfort and the soft tissue has rolled over the nail.

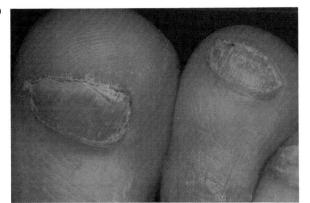

949 Onycholysis. This is caused by the subungual hyperkeratosis that heaps up under the nail. Psoriasis must be excluded.

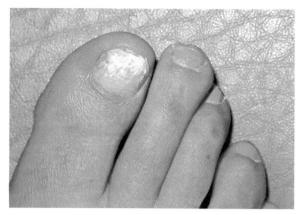

950 Fungus. A crumbling nail or onycholysis may be due to fungal infection of the keratin. Microscopic examination is essential for diagnosis. Most dermatophytes may infect the nails and may be the only sign of fungal infection in an individual. Tinea rubrum and tinea interdigitale may both be found in the toe-nails. Access is gained by the fungus to the nail plate from the free edge or lateral nail fold. It may be seen as a white streak or a crumbling nail.

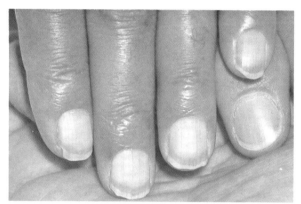

951 White nails—Terry's nails.[23] A white nail bed and a band of normal pink seen distally contrast with the control finger seen adjacent to the patient's fifth finger. The association with disease of the liver is questionable as this change may be found in a quarter of hospital in-patients and in cirrhosis, congestive cardiac failure and diabetes mellitus, as well as in the elderly. The band is due to distal telangiectasia.[24]

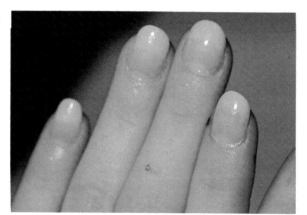

952 and 953 False nails. The unworldly must not fall into the trap of diagnosing white nails when in reality the nails are false ones disguising the bitten nail. This girl compensated by tearing off her toe-nails (**953**) (onychotillomania)!

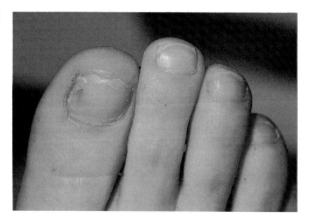

[23]Terry, R. 'White nails in hepatic cirrhosis.' *Lancet*, 1954, **i**: 757–759.
[24]'Terry's nails, Revised definition and new correlations.' *Lancet*, 1984, **i**: 896–899.

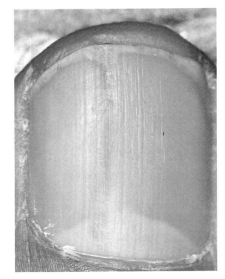

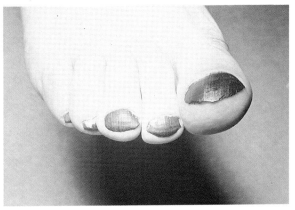

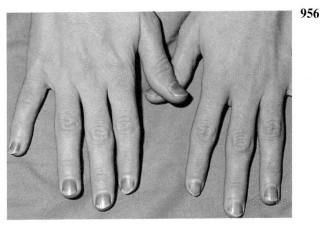

954 Linear naevus. This appearance is due to a junctional naevus in the matrix. It is important to exclude a subungual melanoma and to remember that these naevi may darken in the presence of excess ACTH in the onset of hypo-adrenalcorticalism. In black people the condition may be caused by trauma.

955 and 956 Potassium permanganate nails. Sometimes a diagnostic difficulty may be solved if a careful history is taken. This man, a publican, presented with painful paraesthesiae of the feet which was found to be due to a neuropathy caused by his excess alcohol intake. Liver biopsy showed acute alcoholic hepatitis. The 'nigra-onychia' was due to soaking the feet in potassium permanganate footbaths in an attempt to help the painful tingling. When he decided to seek medical aid he managed to scrub all the stain off the skin, but not from the nails! A similar staining of the nail, but not so intense, is seen with henna (**956**).

Index

Numbers in light type refer to pages; those in **bold** type refer to pictures